AF614777

Update on Bladder Cancer

Edited by Sivapatham Sundaresan

Published in London, United Kingdom

Update on Bladder Cancer
http://dx.doi.org/10.5772/intechopen.102247
Edited by Sivapatham Sundaresan

Contributors
Béla Pikó, Ali Bassam, Anita Kis, Paul Ovidiu Rus-Gal, Ibolya Laczó, Tibor Mészáros, Jaime Villegas O., Emanuel Jeldes, Carlos Contreras, Luis O. Burzio, Verónica Burzio, Vincenzo Borogna, Brent Gilbert, Taryn Naidoo, Azal Al_Rubaeaee, Zahraa Ch. Hameed, Sara Al-Tamemi, Yasukazu Nakanishi, Shugo Yajima, Hitoshi Masuda, Sivapatham Sundaresan, S.K. Lavanya

First published in London, United Kingdom, 2023 by IntechOpen
IntechOpen is the global imprint of INTECHOPEN LIMITED, registered in England and Wales, registration number: 11086078, 5 Princes Gate Court, London, SW7 2QJ, United Kingdom

British Library Cataloguing-in-Publication Data
A catalogue record for this book is available from the British Library

Additional hard and PDF copies can be obtained from orders@intechopen.com

Update on Bladder Cancer
Edited by Sivapatham Sundaresan
p. cm.
Print ISBN 978-1-80356-725-9
Online ISBN 978-1-80356-726-6
eBook (PDF) ISBN 978-1-80356-727-3

For EU product safety concerns:
IN TECH d.o.o., Prolaz Marije Krucifikse Kozulić 3, 51000 Rijeka, Croatia,
info@intechopen.com or visit our website at intechopen.com.

Meet the editor

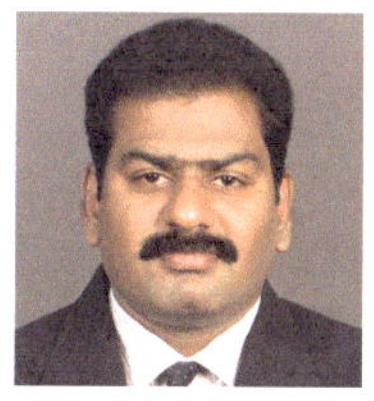

Dr. Sivapatham Sundaresan is an associate professor in the Department of Medical Research, SRM Institute of Science and Technology, India. His research interests include cancer chemoprevention, cancer immunotherapy, and tumor marker detection. His research work includes developing andro/evo-albumin nanoparticles and synthesizing and loading them into polycaprolactone (PCL) scaffolds. He also demonstrated that interferon beta can synergistically work with the chemotherapeutic drug cisplatin for liver, breast, and cervical cancer cells. One of my research disseminated with autophagy proteins Beclin-1, LC3-II and ATG12 and autophagy regulators mTOR, Raptor, p- PRAS40 and Rag C proteins expressions in Head and Neck malignancy distinguishing the tumor types and stages significantly. His recent interests involve investigating the impact of probiotics on the treatment of intestinal toxicity during chemotherapy and their potential to play an adjunct role in Colorectal Cancer. Dr. Sundaresan is a member of the Association of Clinical Biochemists of India and has published many papers in national and international journals.

Contents

Preface

Bladder cancer is the most common malignancy of the urinary tract and one of the most prevalent cancers worldwide. Individualized therapy together with refined surgical techniques and novel systemic as well as intravesical treatment modalities will lead to better oncological outcomes. This book includes six chapters that highlight current research in bladder cancer.

Chapter 1: “Long Non-Coding Mitochondrial RNAs as Novel Molecular Target for Bladder Cancer Treatment”

Chapter 2: “Urobiome and Bladder Cancer”

Chapter 3: “Intracorporeal Urinary Diversion of Robot-Assisted Radical Cystectomy”

Chapter 4: “Review on Bladder Cancer Diagnosis”

Chapter 5: “A Rare but Real Entity: Bladder Neuroendocrine Cancer”

Chapter 6: “Estimation of Some Plant Extract Activity against Bacterial Cystitis Isolated from Urinary Tract Infection”

Sivapatham Sundaresan
Department of Medical Research,
SRM Medical College Hospital and Research Centre,
SRM Institute of Science and Technology,
SRM Nagar, Kattankalathur, Tamil Nadu, India

Chapter 1

Long Non-Coding Mitochondrial RNAs as Novel Molecular Target for Bladder Cancer Treatment

Jaime Villegas O., Vincenzo Borgna, Carlos Contreras, Emanuel Jeldes, Luis O. Burzio and Verónica Burzio

Abstract

Bladder cancer (BC) is the sixth most common cause of cancer; BC risk increases with age and is more common among men than women. Upon diagnosis, the 5-year relative survival rate for patients is approximately 77%. The treatment options available for bladder cancer include chemotherapy, radiation therapy, immunotherapy, targeted therapy, and surgery. Despite the advances in therapeutically novel approaches, BC remains an important problem of public health. Long non-coding RNA (lncRNA) is defined as non-protein-coding RNA molecule longer than 200 nucleotides. Recent findings have highlighted that lncRNA contributes to the regulation of multiple signaling pathways in bladder cancer, suggesting that lncRNA exerts its roles during the biological processes of tumorigenesis, tumor proliferation, differentiation, apoptosis, invasion, migration, and stemness. In our laboratory, we described a family of mitochondrial long non-coding RNAs containing stem-loop structures, named sense and antisense. These transcripts are found outside the organelle, in the cytosol and nucleus in normal and tumor cells, and are differentially expressed according to proliferative status of cells. The antisense transcript seems to be a novel target for BC treatment based in modified antisense oligonucleotides. In this chapter, the novel biology and role of these RNAs as therapeutical targets will be discussed.

Keywords: bladder cancer, mitochondria, antisense oligonucleotides, long non-coding RNAs, bladder cancer treatment

1. Introduction

Bladder cancer (BC) is a complex disease associated with high morbidity and mortality rates if not treated optimally. BC remains the most common malignancy of the urinary tract. In 2018, BC was diagnosed in 549,393 patients and 199,922 succumbed to the disease worldwide [1]. Bladder cancer is the 6th most common cancer in men and 17th most common cancer in women. The incidence of bladder cancer is high in developed countries, and because of rapid industrialization, its worldwide incidence is increasing [2].

A main sign related to the presence of BC is hematuria; however, the final confirmation of the disease must be made using gold standard methodology such as cystoscopy, a procedure that allows a definitive diagnosis and follow-up of the disease. As bladder cancer results in gross or microscopic hematuria, approximately 70 –75% of bladder cancers are diagnosed as non-muscle-invasive bladder cancer (NMIBC) [3]. In the remaining 25–30% of patients, BC has already invaded deeper layers of the bladder wall (MIBC: muscle-invasive disease) or formed metastases. Transurethral resection of the bladder tumor (TURBT) is the mainstay therapy of those with NMIBC, whereas radical removal of the bladder (RC: radical cystectomy) is implemented in those with MIBC [4]. If left without treatment, most patients with MIBC succumb to the disease within 2 years of diagnosis [5]. Therefore, radical cystectomy, followed by meticulous pelvic lymph node dissection, has become the gold standard way of management of muscle-invasive bladder cancer. However, bladder cancer treatment remains a critical issue that requires an urgently new therapeutic approach to fight against this disease.

2. Bladder cancer diagnosis and treatment

There are many approximations to perform bladder cancer diagnosis as cellular morphology analysis and recently the use of novel molecular biomarker as proteins or non-coding RNAs. For instances, urinary cytology evaluates the morphological changes in exfoliated cells from the urinary tract to assess abnormalities [6]. However, the sensitivity of urine cytology varies according to cancer grade. In high-grade urothelial cancer, the sensitivity is as high as 86%, but it is 20–50% in low-grade cancers [3]. It is possible to yield more cellularity, using methods such as catheterization and intravesical washing, but they are limited because of the invasiveness and artifacts caused by the maneuvers [7]. About the urine cytology, a critical issue is that abnormal urine cytology results imply the presence of a tumor, but negative results do not ensure normal conditions. An important problem in urinary cytology corresponds to the cells named borderline: cells that are non-normal but atypical and therefore are confusing for follow-up and diagnosis. Nuclear matrix protein-22 (NMP-22) is involved in the appropriate distribution of chromatin during cellular proliferation and exists at a low level in normal cells but at prominent levels in tumorous conditions [8]. NMP-22 improves the positive predictive value of urine cytology from 30 to 60% [9]. However, due to its variable performance between assays, individuals and even institutions restrict their use in clinics [10].

From a genetic point of view, bladder cancer exhibits aneuploidy of chromosomes (3, 7, and 17) and deletion of the 9p21 locus. This chromosomal profile is the starting point for the development of the commercial kit UroVysion, based on the use of fluorescence *in situ* hybridization (FISH) to detect chromosomal abnormalities [11]. This test was approved by the FDA in 2001 and has been used to diagnose the recurrence of BC from 2001 and to examine gross hematuria from 2005. In addition, it has been suggested that UroVysion FISH be used to judge the response to intravesical BCG therapy. However, one of the big problems about this detection system is its complicated interpretation, which requires expert cytopathology's interpretation and expensive equipment; therefore, the expansion of this diagnostic methodology is restricted at present.

Cancer therapy is an expanding field in search of novel drugs or multimodal approaches to delay or stop the progression of disease. In the case of BC, advanced disease is best treated with systemic cisplatin-based chemotherapy. At present, immunotherapy is emerging as a viable treatment for patients in whom first-line chemotherapy cannot control the disease. Moreover, treatment of patients with advanced disease is undergoing rapid changes as immunotherapy with checkpoint inhibitors, targeted therapies, and antibody–drug conjugates has become an option for certain patients with various stages of disease.

The FDA serially approved the immune checkpoint inhibitors (ICIs) such as atezolizumab, durvalumab, avelumab, pembrolizumab, and nivolumab from 2016 to 2017. Unfortunately, response rates of ICIs result in approximately 20% in patients with advanced BC [12].

This is the beginning of precision medicine for the treatment of patients with this type of malignancy. However, despite the progress in personalized medicine and discovery of novel therapeutic drugs, BC remains an important public health problem. Therefore, new molecular targets are urgently needed for the treatment of this disease.

3. Long non-coding RNAs

Long non-coding RNAs (lncRNAs) belong to a larger and expanding group of non-coding RNAs (ncRNAs) and are classified as 200 nt–100-kb long transcripts, in the absence of open-reading frame [13]. LncRNAs represent a large (>80%) and a very heterogeneous group of ncRNAs, with their expression depending on the tissue and cellular context [14]. These transcripts are indispensable in various cellular processes, including transcription, intracellular trafficking, and chromosome remodeling. In addition, lncRNAs functioning as regulatory factors have been addressed in several complex cellular processes, such as cell death, growth, differentiation, apoptosis, epigenetic regulation, genomic imprinting, alternative splicing, regulation of gene expression at posttranscriptional level, chromatin modification, inflammatory pathologies, and, when deregulated, also in various cancer types [15].

Among the main advantages of lncRNAs that make them suitable as cancer diagnostic and prognostic biomarkers is their high stability while circulating in the body. In addition, lncRNA deregulation in primary tumor tissues is clearly mirrored in various bodily fluids, including whole blood, plasma, urine, saliva, and gastric juice [16].

3.1 Long non-coding RNAs in bladder cancer

In BC, many oncogenic lncRNAs have been shown to be strongly related in bladder carcinogenesis. The lncRNA metastasis-associated lung adenocarcinoma transcript 1 (MALAT1) has been shown to be upregulated in bladder cancer. The effects of MALAT1 knockdown on the inhibition of tumor metastasis have been confirmed in animal models [17, 18], and the experimental evidence indicates that MALAT1 exerts its role in cancer progression and metastasis by enhancing EMT.

Long intergenic non-coding 00346 (LINC00346) silencing can prevent cell proliferation and migration in bladder cancer and can trigger cell cycle arrest and cell apoptosis [19]. The overexpression of lncRNA small nucleolar RNA host gene16 (SNHG16) is significantly correlated with aggressive bladder cancer, and its knockdown can enhance the effect of chemotherapy in bladder cancer cell lines [20]. Terminal differentiation-induced ncRNA (TINCR) has been demonstrated to be upregulated in bladder cancer tissues and cells and participates in cancer development and progression [21].

Silencing of antisense non-coding RNA in the INK4 locus (ANRIL) induces an inhibition of cell proliferation and increase in the cell apoptosis, together with diminished expression of Bcl-2 and elevated expressions of Bax, cytoplasmic cytochrome c, Smac, cleaved caspase-9, caspase-3, and PARP, which are proteins actively involved in apoptosis. *In vivo* studies endorsed the effect of ANRIL silencing in the suppression of tumorigenicity of bladder cancer cells in nude mice [22].

The lncRNA-growth arrest-specific 5 (GAS5) is regarded as a tumor suppressor in bladder cancer because the knockdown of this gene increases bladder cancer cell proliferation, while its forced overexpression inhibits cell proliferation [23]. A recent study has shown that overexpression of GAS5 decreases chemotherapy resistance to doxorubicin in bladder carcinoma [24].

The experimental evidence indicates that lncRNAs can influence oncogenesis and tumor formation in bladder tissues and constitute a novel therapeutical target for diagnosis and treatment.

3.2 A new and exciting family of long non-coding RNAs in bladder cancer: chimeric transcripts

In recent years, a new group of non-coding RNAs have been identified in cancer. These are named fusion genes, which are the consequences of structural rearrangements of the genome as copy number variations, translocations, and inversions, resulting in the concatenation of two different genes or gene fragments [25]. Fusion transcripts or chimeric RNAs that originate from fusion genes are unique to a cancer type, and they are used as novel tools to understand the underlying mechanisms of malignancy and can serve as effective diagnostic and prognostic markers and novel molecular targets [26].

Several groups have shown that chimeric fusion RNAs can be found in various cells and tissues, and some are shown to be the products of intergenic splicing and trans-splicing, instead of chromosomal rearrangement [27, 28]. On the other hand, recent work on RNA trans-splicing [29–31] and intergenic cis-splicing [32] has supported a new paradigm for new and exciting roles of these chimeric RNAs in normal and tumor cell physiology.

Recently, it was described that after an exhaustive analysis of nearly 300 RNA-Seq libraries, covering 30 different non-neoplastic human tissue an cells, including 15 mouse tissues, a large number of chimeric RNAs were found; for instance, 291 chimeric transcripts were seen in more of one sample or tissue, and instead of being transcriptional noise, most of them are functional and translated in chimeric proteins, but interestingly, a large population of fusions may function as non-coding RNAs [33].

In the case of bladder cancer, some chimeric RNAs are being validated in cells and clinical samples; for example, two non-coding RNAs, BCL2L2-PABPN1 and CHFR-GOLGA3, were detected to be expressed significantly higher in bladder cancer samples compared to adjacent normal samples, and these two fusions are generated by cis-splicing between adjacent genes and detected mainly in the fraction of cell nucleus, suggesting a potential long non-coding RNA role in cancer [34]. These novel chimeric RNAs are a new player in the biology of cancer.

"Normal" long non-coding RNAs have been described extensively in association with contrasting functions in bladder cancer; several oncogenic and tumor suppressive lncRNAs have been identified, such as H19, MALAT1, MEG3, SNHG16, TUG1, and

UCA1 [35]. LncRNA expression levels often correlate with prognosis and metastasis formation [36, 37] or occurrence of therapy resistance [38]. In bladder cancer, the upregulation of UCA1 was found to induce epithelial mesenchymal transition (EMT), tumor cell migration, and invasion [39], and it was shown to have a pivotal role in the induction of cisplatin and gemcitabine resistance. Because of their significant role in cancer development, lncRNAs might be potential targets for development of new therapies.

4. Mitochondria as a source of chimeric long non-coding RNAs: novel target for bladder cancer treatment

The mitochondrial genome, unlike the complex nuclear genome, is a compact, circular, and double-stranded DNA encoding only 13 proteins, which are all subunits of the electron transport chain as well as two rRNAs (16S and 12S) and 22 tRNAs required for their translation [40]. Mitochondrial DNA (mtDNA) is composed of heavy (H-strand) and light (L-strand) strands due to the uneven distribution of guanines between DNA strands [41]. In humans, the H-strand of mitochondrial DNA is a template for the transcription of most mitochondrially encoded genes, while the transcription of the complementary L-strand results in the formation of mostly non-coding RNA (ncRNA) [42].

Our laboratory has described a family of chimeric long non-coding RNAs of mitochondrial origin. One of them, named sense non-coding mitochondrial RNA (SncmtRNA), is expressed in both normal proliferating cells and tumor cells. This transcript of 2374 nucleotides contains a long-inverted repeat (IR) linked to the 5′ end of the mature 16S mitochondrial rRNA (16S mtrRNA). The presence of the IR generates a stem-loop structure with an 820-bp double-stranded region and a 40-nt loop [43]. Beside the ScnmtRNA, normal proliferating cells express two novel chimeric RNAs, both containing IRs linked to the 5′ region of the antisense 16S mtRNA transcribed from the L-strand of the mtDNA, named antisense ncmtRNA-1 (ASncmtRNA-1) and ASncmtRNA-2. According to *in situ* hybridization assays, these transcripts show a low level of expression in tumor cells and tumor tissues derived from patients. In contrast, these RNAs are highly expressed in normal proliferating cells [44].

To evaluate the role of these chimeric RNAs, interference assay was made using antisense oligonucleotides targeting both antisense transcripts, using a phosphorothioate oligonucleotide targeting the common loop region of both ASncmtRNAs. We show that the knockdown of the low copy number of ASncmtRNAs in several tumor cell lines induces cell proliferation arrest and cell death mediated by apoptosis without affecting the viability of normal cells. In addition, knockdown of ASncmtRNAs potentiates apoptotic cell death by inhibiting survivin expression, a member of the inhibitor of apoptosis (IAP) family [45].

This molecular approximation suggests us that the ASncmtRNAs are promising targets for cancer therapy, including bladder cancer. Therefore, we evaluated the effects of antisense treatment *in vitro* and *in vivo* in bladder cancer. We found that antisense treatment in three different cell lines, UMUC-3, RT-4, and T-24, induces a strong inhibition of cell proliferation mediated by apoptosis induction. Moreover, the treatment negatively impacts the invasive capacity and spheroid formation of UMUC-3 cells, mediated by the downregulation of N-cadherin and MMP11. This anti-tumoral action was validated in *in vivo* assays using subcutaneous xenograft model and patient-derived xenograft (PDX), where a strong delay of tumor growth was observed [46].

4.1 Putative mechanism of induction of cell death after knockdown of AsmcmtRNAs

As indicated above, knockdown of antisense non-coding mitochondrial RNAs using a complementary oligonucleotide against the loop region results in cell death and apoptosis induction in tumor cells. Recently, we have performed a transcriptomic analysis of changes induced after knockdown of these transcripts in the breast cancer cell line MDA-MB-231. This analysis was performed because we show that ASncmtRNA knockdown induces cell death preceded by proliferative blockage. A partial answer to this cell proliferation block is the fact that knockdown of ASncmtRNAs induces downregulation of some components involved in cell cycle progression and cell survival, as cyclin B1, cyclin D1, CDK1, CDK4, and survivin, with the latter also constituting an essential inhibitor of apoptosis. An interesting effect observed post-treatment was the induction of an increased level of the microRNA hsa-miR-4485-3p. Validation of the target molecule of this miRNA using a mimic shows that in transfected cells the mRNAs of cyclin B1 and D1 are strongly downregulated [47].

Preliminary *in silico* analysis of the affected pathways indicated that proteins involved in cell cycle, apoptosis induction, and cell survival are affected. Moreover, the analysis of the miRNAs that show significant changes in its expression levels shows that some of these small non-coding RNAs have molecular target mRNAs that code for cell cycle checkpoint proteins and cell survival (unpublished results).

These last results constitute an effort to understand the mechanisms underlying the induction of cell death after the knockdown of ASmtncRNAs and sheds light on the role of this family of transcripts in cell cycle progression and tumor biology.

5. Conclusions

Despite the advances of the therapeutic tools developed against bladder cancer, this disease is still a major public health problem, and new molecular targets are required.

Non-coding RNAs are transcripts that do not code for proteins and are involved in the regulation of multiple metabolic pathways in normal cells and tumor cells. Therefore, they constitute a novel family of molecules that may constitute novel therapeutic targets. Chimeric long non-coding RNAs are novel transcripts, and their importance in bladder cancer has recently been evaluated. In this novel field, the mitochondria may play a key role as a source of chimeric transcripts that can constitute new and efficient therapeutic targets. Therefore, the role of these RNAs in the biology of bladder carcinogenesis warrants intensive research to understand their specific role in cancer biology and improve the options for new and effective molecular targets that ensure the efficacy of treatments against this disease.

Acknowledgements

This research was funded by Centro Ciencia & Vida, FB210008, Financiamiento Basal para Centros Científicos y Tecnológicos de Excelencia de ANID, Chile.

Appendices and nomenclature

lncmtRNA	long non-coding mitochondrial ribonucleic acid
SncmtRNA	sense non-coding mitochondrial ribonucleic acid
ASncmtRNA	antisense non-coding mitochondrial ribonucleic acid
BC	bladder cancer
mtDNA	mitochondrial deoxyribonucleic acid
ncRNA	non-coding ribonucleic acid

Author details

Jaime Villegas O.[1,2,3*], Vincenzo Borgna[4,5,6], Carlos Contreras[2], Emanuel Jeldes[1], Luis O. Burzio[2,3] and Verónica Burzio[1,2,3]

1 Centro Científico y Tecnológico de Excelencia Ciencia & Vida, Santiago, Chile

2 School of Medicine Veterinary, Faculty of Life Sciences, Universidad Andrés Bello, Santiago, Chile

3 Andes Biotechnologies Spa, Chile

4 Urology Department, Hospital Barros Luco Trudeau, Chile

5 Faculty of Medicine and Science, Universidad San Sebastian, Chile

6 School of Medicine, Universidad de Santiago de Chile, Santiago, Chile

*Address all correspondence to: jaime.villegas@unab.cl

References

[1] Bray F, Ferlay J, Soerjomataram I, Siegel RL, Torre LA, Jemal A. Global cancer statistics 2018: GLOBOCAN estimates of incidence and mortality worldwide for 36 cancers in 185 countries. CA Cancer Journal of Clinical. 2018;**68**:394-424. DOI: 10.3322/caac.21492

[2] Saginala K, Barsouk A, Aluru JS, Rawla P, Padala SA, Barsouk A. Epidemiology of bladder cancer. Medical Science. 2020;**8**:15-25. DOI: 10.3390/medsci8010015

[3] Zhu CZ, Ting HN, Ng KH, Ong TA. A review on the accuracy of bladder cancer detection methods. Journal of Cancer. 2019;**10**:4038-4044. DOI: 10.7150/jca.28989

[4] Dobruch J, Oszczudłowski M. Bladder cancer: Current challenges and future directions. Medicina. 2021;**57**:749. DOI: org/10.3390/ medicina57080749

[5] Prout GR, Marshall VF. The prognosis with untreated bladder tumors. Cancer. 1956;**3**:551-558. DOI: 10.1002/1097-0142(195605/06)9:3<551:aid-cncr2820090319>3.0.co;2-2

[6] Woldu SL, Bagrodia A, Lotan Y. Guideline of guidelines: Non-muscle-invasive bladder cancer. BJU International. 2017;**119**:371-380. DOI: 10.1111/bju.13760

[7] Sullivan PS, Chan JB, Levin MR, Rao J. Urine cytology and adjunct markers for detection and surveillance of bladder cancer. American Journal of Translational Research. 2010;**2**:412-440

[8] Têtu B. Diagnosis of urothelial carcinoma from urine. Modern Pathology. 2009;**22**:S53-S59. DOI: 10.1038/modpathol.2008.193

[9] Ahn JS, Kim HS, Chang SG, Jeon SH. The clinical usefulness of nuclear matrix Protein-22 in patients with atypical urine cytology. Korean Journal of Urology. 2011;**52**:603-606. DOI: 10.4111/kju.2011.52.9.603

[10] Murakami K, Pagano I, Chen R, Sun Y, Goodison S, Rosser CJ, et al. Influencing factors on the Oncuria urinalysis assay: An experimental model. Diagnostics. 2021;**11**:1023. DOI: 10.3390/diagnostics11061023

[11] Nagai T, Naiki T, Etani T, Iida K, Noda Y, Shimizu N, et al. UroVysion fluorescence in situ hybridization in urothelial carcinoma: A narrative review and future perspectives. Translational Andrology and Urology. 2021;**10**:1908-1917. DOI: 10.21037/tau-201207

[12] Vlachostergios PJ, Jakubowski CD, Niaz MJ, Lee A, Thomas C, Hackett AL, et al. Antibody-drug conjugates in bladder cancer. Bladder Cancer. 2018;**4**:247-259. DOI: 10.3233/BLC-180169

[13] Lee C, Kikyo N. Strategies to identify long noncoding RNAs involved in gene regulation. Cell & Bioscience. 2012;**2**(37):2012. DOI: org/10.1186/2045-3701-2-37

[14] Harrow J, Frankish A, Gonzalez JM, Tapanari E, Diekhans M, Kokocinski F, et al. GENCODE: The reference human genome annotation for the ENCODE project. Genome Research. 2012;**9**:1760-1774. DOI: 10.1101/gr.135350.111

[15] Harries L. Long non-coding RNAs and human disease. Biochemical Society Transactions. 2012;**40**:902-906. DOI: 10.1042/BST20120020

[16] Bolha L, Ravnik-Glavač M, Glavač D. Long noncoding RNAs as biomarkers in cancer. Disease Markers. 2017;**2017**:7243968. DOI: 10.1155/2017/7243968

[17] Fan Y, Shen B, Tan M, Mu X, Qin Y, Zhang F, et al. TGF-βinduced upregulation of malat1 promotes bladder cancer metastasis by associating with suz12. Clinical Cancer Research. 2014;**20**:1531-1541. DOI: 10.1158/1078-0432.CCR-13-1455

[18] Ying L, Chen Q, Wang Y, Zhou Z, Huang Y. upregulated MALAT-1 contributes to bladder cancer cell migration by inducing epithelial-to-mesenchymal transition. Molecular BioSystems. 2012;**8**:2289-2294. DOI: 10.1039/c2mb25070e

[19] Ye T, Ding W, Wang N, Huang H, Pan Y, Wei A. Long noncoding RNAlinc00346 promotes the malignant phenotypes of bladder cancer. Biochemical and Biophysical Research Communications. 2017;**491**:79-84. DOI: 10.1016/j.bbrc.2017.07.045

[20] Zhu Y, Yu M, Li Z, Kong C, Bi J, Li J, et al. ncRAN, a newly identified long noncoding RNA, enhances human bladder tumor growth, invasion, and survival. Urology. 2011;**77**:510-511

[21] Chen Z, Liu Y, He A, Li J, Chen M, Zhan Y, et al. Theophylline controllable RNAi-based genetic switches regulate expression of lncRNATINCR and malignant phenotypes in bladder cancer cells. Scientific Reports. 2016b;**6**:30798

[22] Taheri M, Davood Omrani M, Ghafouri-Fard S. Long non-coding RNA expression in bladder cancer. Biophysical Reviews. 2018;**2018**:1205-1213. DOI: /10.1007/s12551-017-0379-y

[23] Cao Q, Wang N, Qi J, Gu Z, Shen H. Long non-coding RNAGAS5 acts as a tumor suppressor in bladder transitional cell carcinoma via regulation of chemokine (C-C motif) ligand 1 expression. Molecular Medicine Reports. 2016;**13**:27-34. DOI: 10.3892/mmr.2015.4503

[24] Zhang H, Guo Y, Song Y. Shang C (2017) long noncoding RNA GAS5 inhibits malignant proliferation and chemotherapy resistance to doxorubicin in bladder transitional cell carcinoma. Cancer Chemotherapy and Pharmacology. 2017;**79**:49-55. DOI: 10.1007/s00280-016-3194-4

[25] Inaki K, Hillmer AM, Ukil L, Yao F, Woo XY, Vardy LA, et al. Transcriptional consequences of genomic structural aberrations in breast cancer. Genome Research. 2011;**21**:676-687. DOI: 10.1101/gr.113225.110

[26] Mertens F, Johansson B, Fioretos T, Mitelman F. The emerging complexity of gene fusions in cancer. Nature Reviews. Cancer. 2015;**15**:371-381. DOI: 10.1038/nrc3947

[27] Wu CS, Yu CY, Chuang CY, Hsiao M, Kao CF, Kuo HC, et al. Integrative transcriptome sequencing identifies trans-splicing events with important roles in human embryonic stem cell pluripotency. Genome Research. 2014;**24**:25-36. DOI: 10.1101/gr.159483.113

[28] Chase A, Ernst T, Fiebig A, Collins A, Grand F, Erben P, et al. TFG, a target of chromosome translocations in lymphoma and soft tissue tumors, fuses to GPR128 in healthy individuals. Haematologica. 2010;**2010**(95):20-26. DOI: 10.3324/haematol.2009.011536

[29] Yuan H, Qin F, Movassagh M, Park H, Golden W, Xie Z, et al. A chimeric RNA characteristic of rhabdomyosarcoma in normal

myogenesis process. Cancer Discovery. 2013;**12**:1394-1403. DOI: 10.1158/2159-8290.CD-13-0186

[30] Li H, Wang J, Mor G, Sklar J. A neoplastic gene fusion mimics trans-splicing of RNAs in normal human cells. Science. 2008;**321**:1357-1361. DOI: 10.1126/science.1156725

[31] Finta C, Zaphiropoulos PG. Intergenic mRNA molecules resulting from trans splicing. The Journal of Biological Chemistry. 2002;**277**:5882-5890. DOI: 10.1074/jbc.M109175200

[32] Qin F, Song Z, Babiceanu M, Song Y, Facemire L, Singh R, et al. Discovery of CTCF-Sensitive cis-spliced fusion RNAs between adjacent genes in human prostate cells. PloS Genetics. 2015;**11**:e1005001

[33] Babiceanu M, Qin F, Xie Z, Jia Y, Lopez K, Janus N, et al. Recurrent chimeric fusion RNAs in non-cancer tissues and cells. Nucleic Acids Research. 2016;**44**:2859-2872. DOI: 10.1093/nar/gkw032

[34] Zhu D, Singh S, Chen X, Zheng Z, Huang J, Lin T, et al. The landscape of chimeric RNAs in bladder urothelial carcinoma. The International Journal of Biochemistry & Cell Biology. 2019;**110**:50-58. DOI: 10.1016/j.biocel.2019.02.007

[35] Martens-Uzunova ES, Böttcher R, Croce CM, Jenster G, Visakorpi T, Calin GA. Long noncoding RNA in prostate, bladder, and kidney cancer. European Urology. 2014;**65**:1140-1151. DOI: 10.1016/j.eururo.2013.12.003

[36] Jadaliha M, Zong X, Malakar P, Ray T, Singh DK, Freier SM, et al. Functional and prognostic significance of long non-coding RNA MALAT1 as a metastasis driver in ER negative lymph node negative breast cancer. Oncotarget. 2016;**7**:40418-40436. DOI: 10.18632/oncotarget.9622

[37] Prensner JR, Iyer MK, Sahu A, Asangani IA, Cao Q, Patel L, et al. The long noncoding RNA SChLAP1 promotes aggressive prostate cancer and antagonizes the SWI/SNF complex. Nature Genetics. 2013;**45**:1392-1398. DOI: 10.1038/ng.2771

[38] Teschendorff AE, Lee SH, Jones A, Fiegl H, Kalwa M, Wagner W, et al. HOTAIR and its surrogate DNA methylation signature indicate carboplatin resistance in ovarian cancer. Genome Medicine. 2015;**7**:108. DOI: 10.1186/s13073-015-0233-4

[39] Xue M, Pang H, Li X, Li H, Pan J, Chen W. Long non-coding RNA urothelial cancer-associated 1 promotes bladder cancer cell migration and invasion by way of the has-miR-145-ZEB1/2-FSCN1 pathway. Cancer Science. 2016;**107**:18-27. DOI: 10.1111/cas.12844

[40] Smeitink J, van den Heuvel L, DiMauro S. The genetics and pathology of oxidative phosphorylation. Nature Reviews. Genetics. 2001;**2**:342-352. DOI: 10.1038/35072063

[41] Anderson S, Bankier AT, Barrell BG, de Bruijn MH, Coulson AR, Drouin J, et al. Sequence and organization of the human mitochondrial genome. Nature. 1981;**9**(290):457-465. DOI: 10.1038/290457a0

[42] Attardi G, Chomyn A, King MP, Kruse B, Polosa PL, Murdter NN. Regulation of mitochondrial gene expression in mammalian cells. Biochemical Society Transactions. 1990;**18**:509-513. DOI: 10.1042/bst0180509J

[43] Villegas J, Burzio V, Villota C, Landerer E, Martinez R, Santander M,

et al. Expression of a novel non-coding mitochondrial RNA in human proliferating cells. Nucleic Acids Research. 2007;**35**:7336-7347. DOI: 10.1093/nar/gkm863

[44] Burzio VA, Villota C, Villegas J, Landerer E, Boccardo E, Villa LL, et al. Expression of a family of noncoding mitochondrial RNAs distinguishes normal from cancer cells. Proceedings of the National Academy Science USA. 2009;**106**:9430-9434. DOI: 10.1073/pnas.0903086106

[45] Vidaurre S, Fitzpatrick C, Burzio VA, Briones M, Villota C, Villegas J, et al. Down-regulation of the antisense mitochondrial non-coding RNAs (ncRNAs) is a unique vulnerability of cancer cells and a potential target for cancer therapy. The Journal of Biological Chemistry. 2014;**289**:27182-27198. DOI: 10.1074/jbc.M114.558841

[46] Borgna V, Lobos-González L, Guevara F, Landerer E, Bendek M, Ávila R, et al. Targeting antisense mitochondrial noncoding RNAs induces bladder cancer cell death and inhibition of tumor growth through reduction of survival and invasion factors. Journal of Cancer. 2020;**11**:1780-1791. DOI: 10.7150/jca.38880

[47] Fitzpatrick C, Bendek MF, et al. Mitochondrial ncRNA targeting induces cell cycle arrest and tumor growth inhibition of MDA-MB-231 breast cancer cells through reduction of key cell cycle progression factors. Cell Death & Disease. 2019;**10**:423. DOI: 10.1038/s41419-019-1649-3

Chapter 2

Urobiome and Bladder Cancer

Brent Gilbert and Taryn Naidoo

Abstract

Microbiome studies, fueled by the availability of high-throughput DNA-based techniques, have shown that microbiome alterations is associated with human disease including cancer. Traditionally, bladder epithelium and urine have been considered sterile in healthy individuals. This was based primarily on microbiological urine cultures, best suited for detecting aerobic, fast-growing uropathogens. Microbiome and new culturing techniques have shown that urine is not sterile but contains distinct commensal microorganisms and that alterations in commensal bladder microbes is associated with bladder cancer. This chapter focuses on identifying commensal and tumorigenic bladder bacteria, the alterations that occur in bladder cancer and impact on current treatments.

Keywords: bladder cancer, microbiome, urine cultures, schistosomiasis, urobiome

1. Introduction

The human microbiome consists of all bacteria, viral and fungal genetic material that coexists within our body [1, 2]. The microbiome is involved in a number of complex interactions with host cells, metabolic processes and the immune system which can culminate in suppression or enhancement of cancer [1]. The microbiome is not a stable entity but changes with time as people age and can be directly altered by a number of environmental and host factors [1]. To better understand the human microbiome a concerted international effort began to catalog the core microbial composition of healthy human body in the Human Microbiome Project (HMP; https://commonfund.nih.gov/hmp/) [2].

As a result of this endeavor microbial changes have been shown to be associated with multiple malignancies including colorectal, gastric, lung and breast [3]. Originally the urinary microbiota was not included in the HMP [2]. Historically it has been taught that the bladder and urine are sterile. This concept dates back to early experiments by Louis Pasteur who found that urine contained in sealed vials did not become cloudy – suggesting a lack of bacteria [4]. Over subsequent decades culturing techniques improved but only enabled detection of a limited number of bacteria, mainly aerobic, fast-growing bacteria such as *Escherichia coli* [4]. Anaerobic, slow-growing bacteria with complex nutritional needs were not detected using traditional culturing techniques. Analysis of traditional culturing techniques disregarded low bacterial yields as contaminates which further perpetuated the belief that urine was sterile and any bacteria grown must be a contaminate or an invading pathogen from genital, skin or gastrointestinal source [4].

This presumption came into refute ten years ago when it was shown that through next generation sequencing techniques (NGS) using 16 s ribosomal RNA PCR and whole genome shotgun sequencing that urine is not sterile but replete with various microorganisms and biofilms [5]. These findings found that the healthy human bladder is colonized by a living, dynamic environment of changing microbiota. Many of the microorganisms characterized in urine were not known to cause symptomatic urinary tract infections (UTI) and are believed to be commensals. Utilization of NGS has enabled identification of new commensal and emerging uropathogens [5–8].

A drawback of NGS techniques is its inability to show the viability of bacteria identified. As a result traditional urine culturing techniques have improved to broaden the range of identifiable bacteria [9]. The use of expanded quantitative urine culture (EQUC) protocols have been incorporated into routine practice [9]. Compared to traditional culturing techniques, EQUC analyses a larger volume of urine. Samples are inoculated into multiple growth mediums and are incubated for longer periods of time under aerobic and anaerobic conditions [9]. The combined use of NGS and EQUC strategies has improved detection of urinary microbes, but distinguishing commensal from potential uropathogen continues to be defined.

The collection of microbes in the urine has been coined the urobiome and imbalances in a healthy urobiome is referred to as dysbiosis. Urinary dysbiosis is believed to contribute to a number of urological conditions including interstitial cystitis, chronic lower urinary tract symptoms and bladder cancer [10].

2. The Urobiome

2.1 Urine sampling

Urine sampling methods can dramatically impact bacterial detection and must be taken into consideration when trying to establish the normal urine microbiome. Many studies have used midstream urine samples which is not a sterile collection method. It has the potential to contain contaminants from peri-urethral or genital tract and may mislead proper characterization of the urine microbiome in favor of urogenital microbiome [8, 11]. Given anatomic differences between men and women this also poses variation of the sources of contamination. Transurethral catheters reduces the risk of contamination but it is invasive and can still potentially result in urethral bacterial contamination during catheter insertion [12]. Collecting urine via suprapubic aspiration is regarded as the most accurate method and produces less risk contamination, however one study has shown that urine microbiota obtained via transurethral catheter or suprapubic aspiration produces similar results [5]. Regardless of the specimen collection technique the urobiome has been shown to change considerably based on age, gender, race and geographic distribution [5, 8].

2.2 Defining the healthy Urobiome

Compared with vaginal and gut microbiota, the urinary microbiota has significantly less biomass. For instance, female urine is estimated to contain 10^4-10^5 colony forming units (CFU) /mL compared to 10^{12} CFU in feces [7]. There have been 562 documented species in urine and there is significant overlap with gut (64% similar) and vaginal (31% similar) microbes such that only 185 species identified are unique to urine [13, 14].

The urobiome predominantly consists of bacteria and to a lesser extent fungi, viruses and arachae. Taxonomically, microbes are classified according to phyla, classes, orders, families, genera, and species. The phyla taxa of the urobiome is similar for men and women with the majority of bacteria belonging to the phyla Firmicutes (65% in males vs. 73% in females). The other predominate phyla include Actinobacteria (15% in males, vs. 19% in females), Bacteroidetes (10% in males vs. 3% in females) and Proteobacteria (8% in males vs. 3% in females) and 2-3% is spread across a number of low abundant phyla [11]. Urine from healthy men and women share a number of common genera with the three most prominent being Lactobacillus, Corynebacterium and Streptococcus [6, 8]. There are, however, distinct differences between the female and male urobiome.

2.3 The female Urobiome

Given the anatomical proximity between the bladder and vagina, microbial colonization of the bladder may originate or be interconnected with the vaginal microbiota. Same donor studies have revealed significant overlap of uropathogens and commensals residing in vaginal and vesicle microbiotas [15, 16]. Similar organisms included *E. coli, Streptococcus anginosus*, *Lactobacillus iners*, *Lactobacillus crispatus* and the operative taxonomic units (OTU) of *Gardnerella*, *Prevotella*, *Ureaplasma* [15, 16].

Lactobacillus is the most abundant genus found in the female urobiome and has significantly higher levels than those seen in men [7, 8, 11, 17]. Decreased levels of Lactobacillus have been associated with women of advanced age and pathological states such as UTI and Bladder cancer (BCa) [8, 18–21]. However reduced levels of *Lactobacillus* is not always a predictor of health as increased *Lactobacillus gasseri* is associated with urge urinary incontinence (UUI). *Gardnerella*, the second most abundant genera in the urobiome is also a genitourinary microbe. Gardnerella genus primarily consists of *Gardnerella vaginalis* and is a potential UTI causing uropathogen [7].

2.4 The male Urobiome

The male urobiome is less studied than the female urobiome and samples are often obtained from mid-stream urine which are prone to contamination [6]. The male microbiome is predominantly characterized by *Corynebacterium* [8] and *Streptococcus* [11] and contains less abundant *Lactobacillus* compared to women [7, 8, 11, 17]. *Pseudomonas* has also only been identified healthy men and *Staphylococcus haemolyticus* appears to have higher relative abundance in men than women [22].

2.5 Age related Urobiome changes

A number of bacteria have been shown to decrease with age. In women these include *Lactobacillus*, *Bifidobacteria*, *Sneathia*, *Shuttlewothia* and *Bacillus* [16, 19, 23]. These changes are thought to coincide with a reduction in estrogen associated with menopause. Conversely post-menopausal women show an increased relative abundance of *Mobiluncus*, *Oligella* and *Porphyromonas* [23]. Regardless of gender, individuals over 70 years have increased levels of *Jonquetella*, *Parvimonas*, *Proteiniphilum* and *Saccharofermentans* [6, 23].

2.6 The urine Virome

A number of human and bacteriophage viruses have been characterized in healthy urine specimens. Human viruses such as BK and JC polyomavirus, Herpesvirus,

Adenovirus and Anellovirus are known to reside in human urine [22, 24, 25]. These viruses have the potential to cause UTIs in immunocompromised hosts and have been associated with overactive bladders [24, 26]. Human papillomaviruses (HPVs) have also been detected in voided urine and bladder tissue [27, 28]. High risk HPV genotypes associated with cervical cancer have also been attributed to condyloma acuminatum of the bladder but there has been no direct correlation with bladder specific cancer [29, 30]. Urine may serve as a potential reservoir for local transmission of human viruses.

The vast majority of viruses in urine are bacteriophages. These viruses infect urinary bacteria such as *Lactobacillus*, *Gardnerella*, *E. coli*, *Enterococcus*, *Pseudomonas* and *Staphylococcus* [26]. Bacteriophages have been found in the urinary microbiota of both healthy women and women with UTIs [26]. Complete cataloging of bacteriophages in the urinary virome is ongoing and their contribution to urinary dysbiosis and potential association with bladder cancer is being defined [26].

2.7 The fungal and archaea Urobiome

It is difficult to ascertain if fungal and archaea cultures are naturally occurring in the urobiome or whether they are a source of contamination [31]. Midstream urine has the potential to become contaminated by nearby genitals which is known to contain fungal cultures. However, catheterized urine samples from middle aged female patients has shown to contain *Candida* spp. [7]. To date, the only archaea to be associated with urine is *Methanobrevibacter smithii* - a well-studied normal organism of the gut microbiota that it is associated with Enterobacteriaceae UTIs [32].

3. The Urobiome and bladder cancer

The relationship between the urine microbiome and cancer remains to be defined. It is possible that the urinary microbiome influences the development or progression of bladder cancer or alternatively bladder cancer influences the diversity, composition and abundance of bladder microbes.

One hypothesis is that the bladder microbiome alters the extracellular matrix which may inhibit or promote inflammation and urothelial cell carcinogenesis. When the urothelial barrier is breached, inflammatory responses promoted by opportunistic invasion of resident microbes may promote tumorigenesis. Biofilms, are microbial communities embedded in a biopolymer matrix. They are highly resistant to antibiotics and host immune responses and therefore can potentiate and propagate chronic inflammation. Bacterial biofilms have been shown to play a role in the development of a number of cancers including BCa [33]. Biofilms promote bacterial adherence, urothelial cell injury and correlates with a higher risk of developing BCa [33].

3.1 Schistosomiasis and bladder cancer

In North America and Europe approximately 90% of BCa are urothelial cell carcinoma (UCC) [34]. In Africa and the Middle East UCC bladder cancer represents 53-69% of cases and 10-40% of cases are squamous cell carcinoma (SCC) due to endemic infections of Schistosoma species [35].

Schistosoma haematobium and *Schistosoma mansoni* are common parasitic flukes that are found in fresh water primarily in sub-Sarahan Africa, South America and sporadically in the Middle East [36]. The parasites enter the urinary tract via exposure to fresh water and lay eggs which cause inflammation and scarring of the genitourinary tract [36]. This chronic inflammation leads to squamous cell metaplasia of the urothelium and over time results in squamous cell carcinoma of the bladder [36].

The exact mechanism by which Schistosoma ova causes SCC is unclear but two factors are suspected. Firstly squamous epithelium shows greater proliferation compared to urothelial cells and hence the higher turnover of cells increase the spontaneous risk of genetic alterations that can cause cancer [37]. Secondly, chronic inflammation and exposure to environmental agents can combine to generate genotoxic urinary substances such as N-butyl-N-(4-hydroxybutyl) nitrosamine (N-Nitrosamines). N-Nitrosamines are generated in very high levels in the urine of *Schistosomiasis* patients and are known carcinogenic compounds [38]. Chronic schistosomiasis leads predominantly to SCC rather than UCC with approximately 70% of infected patients developing SCC; however many patients will have both SCC and UCC [39]. Interestingly, alterations in the urobiome may influence *Schistosomiasis* related bladder cancer. Individuals infected with Schistosomiasis and had urine colonized with *Fusobacterium, Sphingobacterium* or *Enterococcus* were more likely to progress to bladder cancer [40]. It is suggested that strains of bacteria which mediate the formation of N-nitrosamines contribute to schistosomiasis-induced bladder cancer [40].

3.2 Urothelial cancer and the Urobiome

The urobiome and its role in bladder cancer is an emerging field of investigation and the interpretation of findings is often difficult to appreciate given the various host, environmental and sampling factors that contribute and can significantly alter the composition of the urobiome. There is also a great deal of variation when it comes to specimen processing, sequencing targets, taxonomy assignment databases and statistical analysis performed. These issues must be taken into consideration when interpreting findings. Most of our understanding so far regarding the urobiome in bladder cancer is generated from retrospective cohort and case control studies. There have been very few prospective or higher level research studies to date [41].

Bacterial diversity within a sample is quantified by several statistical methods and is expressed as alpha-diversity (α-diversity). Whereas beta-diversity (β-diversity) is a measure of diversity between two environments ie; bladder cancer vs. no cancer. So far there is no consensus regarding BCa urine/tissue having greater or less bacterial diversity or species richness [41]. However there are certain genus/species which have been reported to be more common in BCa specimens (**Table 1**).

3.3 Microbial changes in urothelial cancer

A number of studies have identified higher abundances of **Acinetobacter** genus in tissue and urine of bladder cancer patients [20, 21, 42, 43]. **Acinetobacter** is a complex genus consisting of gram-negative, anaerobic, biofilm forming species [44]. **Acinetobacter** is capable of adhering, degrading and invading urothelial barriers. This allows it to evade antibiotics and host immune responses and possibly promote carcinogenesis directly through urothelial injury or alterations of cell-cycle proliferation, or indirectly enabling invasion of other opportunistic tumorigenic uropathogens [44, 45]. **Actinomyces** genus is a common urogenital commensal that is often seen in women and has the potential to cause suppurative and granulomatous opportunistic infections. *Actinomyces*, in particular *A. europaeus,* is increased in the urine of BCa

Genera	Sample	Bladder Cancer Trend	Known functional effect
Acinetobacter	Urine Tissue	↑ ↑	Biofilm forming genus Invasive pathogen that can degrade phospholipid membranes Associated with urothelial cancer in other species
Actinomyces (*A. europaeus*)	Urine	↑	Opportunistic uropathogen
Actinotignum	Urine	↑	Opportunistic uropathogen elevated in women
Anaerococcus	Urine	↑	Biofilm producer Opportunistic uropathogen Extracellular matrix remodeling
Aeromonas	Urine	↑	Secrete extracellular proteases
Tepidomonas	Urine	↑	Secrete extracellular proteases
Pseudomonas	Urine	↑	Secrete extracellular proteases Secretes anti-tumor exotoxin-A immunotoxin Elevated in BCG Responders
Burkholderia	Urine Tissue	↑ ↑	Inhibits tumorigenesis by blocking CTLA-4 signaling
Sphingomonas	Urine Tissue	↑	Degrades aromatic compounds
Escherichia-Shigella	Urine Tissue	↓ ↑	Uropathogen Secretes genotoxic colibactin toxin Elevated in BCG responders
Klebsiella	Tissue	↑	Uropathogen Secretes genotoxic colibactin toxin Elevated in BCG responders
Lactobacillus	Urine Tissue	↓ ↓	Probiotic with Anti-tumor properties Secretes lactic acid and H2O2 Competitively excludes uropathogens Increases effectiveness of epirubicin
Bifidobacterium	Urine	↓	Induces apoptosis via multiple pathways
Roseomonas	Urine	↓	Improves epithelial barriers Suppresses *S. Aureus* Immunomodulation through lipid mediated TNFa-receptor signaling
Corynebacterium	Urine	↑ and ↓	Opportunistic uropathogen Hydrolyzes lipids yielding anti-bacterial free fatty acids.
Veillonella	Urine IDC Urine	↓ ↑	Utilizes lactic acid produced by Lactobacillus Reduces nitrate levels by converting it to nitrite
Streptococcus	Urine	↑ and ↓	Large genus with multiple species Species have tumorigenic and anti-tumorigenic potentials

IDC – indwelling catheter; BCG – Bacille Calmette-Guerin; TNFα – Tumor Necrosis Factor α; CTLA-4 -Cytotoxic T-lymphocyte associated protein 4.

Table 1.
Summary of genera that have been identified in more than one study and implicated in attenuation or progression of bladder cancer.

patients [18]. **Actinotignum**, an Actinomyces-like organism is a urine commensal and opportunistic uropathogen that was only elevated in female BCa patients [46]. *Anaerococcus*, *Tepidomonas and Pseudomonas* are elevated in voided BCa urine they and can induce inflammation and remodeling of the extracellular matrix (ECM) which provides access to the suburothelial space for opportunistic tumorigenic uropathogens and may contribute to BCa onset, progression and relapse [42, 47, 48]. *Aeromonas*, *Tepidomonas* and *Pseudomonas* secrete extracellular proteases which disrupts the ECM [42, 48]. **Pseudomonas** may also have anti-tumor potential via the production of an exotoxin-A immunotoxin which shows specific and efficacious anti-tumor cytoxocity [49]. To further support anti-tumor properties of *Pseudomonas* it is elevated in the urine of Bacille Calmette-Guerin (BCG) responders compared to BCG non-responders [47]. *Burkholderia* is a urinary commensal that is increased in BCa tissue and urine [47, 50]. Its role in BCa is unknown but it may inhibit tumorigenesis by blocking CTLA-4 signaling [51]. *Sphingomonas* is elevated in BCa tissue and urine and known to degrade carcinogenic aromatic compounds [20, 21, 42, 43, 52].

Corynebacterium is an abundant urinary commensal that is elevated in male urine and reported to be elevated in BCa urine by most studies [43, 50, 53, 54]. When detected in BCa urine it has been associated with high grade NMBC and MBC [8, 53, 54]. *Corynebacterium* species hydrolyze lipids and release free fatty acids with anti-bacterial activity and are also potential opportunistic uropathogens [55]. The role of *Corynebacterium* in the urobiome and possible contribution to BCa is not known. It is unclear if *Eschericihia-Shigella* and *Klebsiella* genus are elevated in BCa [20, 21, 50, 56, 57]. *Eschericihia-Shigella* and *Klebsiella* are uropathogens capable of influencing tumorigenesis by producing genotoxic colibactin; a toxin that induces DNA strand breaks resulting in genomic instability [58]. *Eschericihia-Shigella* is also elevated in BCG responder urine which may indicate that certain bacteria may be needed to be present to prime the immune response for optimal BCG effect [56].

The majority of bacteria that are decreased in BCa tend to beneficial. *Lactobacillus* is a large genus that contributes significantly to the urine commensal population [8, 11]. *Lactobacillus* is urogenital commensal that is found in greater numbers in women compared to men and reduces post-menopause [23]. These microbes play an important role in regulating UTIs through the production of lactic acid and hydrogen peroxide, colonizing resistance and competitively excluding pathogens [59]. The protective role of *Lactobacillus* may translate into reduced tumorigenesis which may help to explain the sex-disparity of bladder cancer [60]. *Bifidobacterium* [18] has been shown to induce apoptosis through intrinsic and extrinsic pathways that involves increasing expression of Fas, FasL, Cyt-C, Caspase-3, Caspase-9 and lowering cancer proliferation proteins such as PCNA, PFK-B, HKK-1, PKM2 [61]. *Roseomonas* is an immunomodulation genus that can improve epithelial barriers and suppresses competing bacteria such as *Staphylococcus aureus* through lipid mediated TNFα- receptor signaling [62].

Veillonella and *Streptococcus* genus are both urinary commensals that have protective potentials which have been shown to be decreased and increased in BCa [18, 43, 47, 54, 56, 57]. *Veillonella* is a probiotic that is capable of using lactic acid produced by Lactobacillus and converting nitrates to nitrites [63]. Higher nitrate levels are thought to contribute to N-nitrosamines formation and increased risk of bladder cancer [64] *Streptococcus* is a large genus which contains a number of species with tumorigenic and anti-tumorigenic potentials [65, 66]. Further investigation at the species level is needed to clarify the role that Streptococcus plays in BCa.

4. The Urobiome and bladder cancer treatment

4.1 Probiotics

Before the microbiome era researchers were aware that oral administration of probiotic bacteria could potentially reduce incidence and recurrence of bladder cancer [67–69]. Specifically, *Lactobacillus casei* and *Lactobacillus rhamnosus* were shown to have cytotoxic effect on BCa cells and inhibited BCa growth. The mechanism may be propagated through NK cell activity but this is not known for sure [70]. A randomized controlled trial compared standard intravesical epirubicin alone with epirubicin plus one year oral intake of *L. casei* strain Shirota in patients who had undergone resection of intermediate-risk NMIBC. A statistically significant 15% absolute reduction in long-term tumor recurrence was seen in the group that received the oral probiotic. However the dropout rate of the probiotic group was 3.5 times the control group and this called into question the reliability of this study [71]. Given that there is renewed interest in microbial influence in BCa and we have new tools to evaluate the microbiome these studies may need to be re-investigated.

4.2 Bacille Calmette-Guerin (BCG) treatment

Intravesical BCG instillations have been a mainstay of adjuvant therapy for high and intermediate risk of non-muscle invasive bladder cancer (NMIBC). BCG failure leading to disease recurrence and progression remains a significant clinical issue. Recent microbiome research has shown that *Escherichia-Shigella*, *Pseudomonas*, and *Serratia* were significantly more abundant in the urine of BCG responsive patients compared to non-responders [56]. The belief is that uropathogenic bacteria is needed to help prime the immune directed response of BCG [72].

The complete mechanism by which BCG controls BCa proliferation still remains unclear. However, BCG is believed to bind fibronectin sites on the urothelial wall and become internalized through RAS and PI3K-PTEN dependent micropinocytosis process. The tumor-specific immune response increases in intensity over the course of the treatment period. A number of urinary microbes can bind fibronectin and have the potential to out-compete BCG for fibronectin binding and attenuate BCG efficacy. One such microbe is *L. iners* which is predominantly found in females and is shown to preferably bind fibronectin and decrease BCG efficacy [73]. Screening urine microbiome and targeting fibronectin binding microbes ahead of BCG treatment may lead to improved treatment outcomes.

4.3 The Urobiome and immunotherapy

The role of the microbiome may extend to advanced BCa disease management. Immunotherapy agents, particularly those utilizing the PD-1/PD-L1 axis have seen increased use in advanced BCa. The efficacy of these agents have been associated with composition of the gut microbiome. It is plausible that the composition of the urobiome may also influence the response of anti-PD1/PDL1 therapy. It has been reported that antibiotic use within one month of starting atezolizumab is associated with reduced overall survival in locally advanced and metastatic platinum-refractory BCa treated by atezolizumab [74]. An additional study has also shown that antibiotic use during pembrolizumab neoadjuvant immunotherapy in MIBC was associated with greater relapse and poorer outcomes [75].

5. Conclusion

The dogma that urine is sterile is no longer acceptable as recent technological advances have shown that urine contains a number of commensal microbes. However, there is still much to learn about the urobiome regarding its composition and function during homeostasis and disease. A number of cross-sectional and case–control studies have identified changes in the urobiome associated with bladder cancer. However, further research using appropriate confounding controls and employing multi-omic approaches is required to clarify the implications of these taxonomic differences and their role in bladder cancer with the hope of establishing diagnostic or prognostic microbial markers and improved therapeutic modalities and outcomes.

Acknowledgements

The authors would like to express a special thanks to the following people for their inspiration and continued support throughout this academic endeavor. Dr. Gerard Kaiko, Dr. Stephen Smith, Dr. Peter Wark, Dr. Candace Naidoo, Mrs. Kathleen Gilbert.

Author details

Brent Gilbert[1,2*] and Taryn Naidoo[2]

1 The University of Newcastle School of Medicine, Newcastle NSW, Australia

2 Surgical Sciences Department, Hunter New England Health, John Hunter Hospital, Newcastle, NSW, Australia

*Address all correspondence to: brentgilbert@gmail.com; brent.gilbert@health.nsw.gov.au

References

[1] Grice EA, Segre JA. The human microbiome: Our second genome. Annual Review of Genomics and Human Genetics. 2012;**13**:151-170

[2] Human Microbiome Project Consortium. Structure, function and diversity of the healthy human microbiome. Nature. 2012;**486**(7402):207-214

[3] Knippel RJ, Drewes JL, Sears CL. The cancer microbiome: Recent highlights and knowledge gaps. Cancer Discovery. 2021;**11**(10):2378-2395

[4] Thomas-White K, Brady M, Wolfe AJ, Mueller ER. The bladder is not sterile: History and current discoveries on the urinary microbiome. Current Bladder Dysfunction Report. 2016;**11**(1):18-24

[5] Wolfe AJ, Toh E, Shibata N, Rong R, Kenton K, Fitzgerald M, et al. Evidence of uncultivated bacteria in the adult female bladder. Journal of Clinical Microbiology. 2012;**50**(4):1376-1383

[6] Lewis DA, Brown R, Williams J, White P, Jacobson SK, Marchesi JR, et al. The human urinary microbiome; bacterial DNA in voided urine of asymptomatic adults. Frontiers in Cellular and Infection Microbiology. 2013;**3**:41

[7] Pearce MM, Hilt EE, Rosenfeld AB, Zilliox MJ, Thomas-White K, Fok C, et al. The female urinary microbiome: A comparison of women with and without urgency urinary incontinence. MBio. 2014;**5**(4):e01283-e01214

[8] Fouts DE, Pieper R, Szpakowski S, Pohl H, Knoblach S, Suh MJ, et al. Integrated next-generation sequencing of 16S rDNA and metaproteomics differentiate the healthy urine microbiome from asymptomatic bacteriuria in neuropathic bladder associated with spinal cord injury. Journal of Translational Medicine. 2012;**10**:174

[9] Price TK, Dune T, Hilt EE, Thomas-White KJ, Kliethermes S, Brincat C, et al. The clinical urine culture: Enhanced techniques improve detection of clinically relevant microorganisms. Journal of Clinical Microbiology. 2016;**54**(5):1216-1222

[10] Shoemaker R, Kim J. Urobiome: An outlook on the metagenome of urological diseases. Investigative and Clinical Urology. 2021;**62**(6):611-622

[11] Modena BD, Milam R, Harrison F, Cheeseman JA, Abecassis MM, Friedewald JJ, et al. Changes in urinary microbiome populations correlate in kidney transplants with interstitial fibrosis and tubular atrophy documented in early surveillance biopsies. American Journal of Transplantation. 2017;**17**(3):712-723

[12] al AHSe. Laboratory diagnosis of urinary tract infections using diagnostics tests in adult patients. International. Journal of Research in Medical Sciences. 2014;**2**(2):415-421

[13] Morand A, Cornu F, Dufour JC, Tsimaratos M, Lagier JC, Raoult D. Human bacterial repertoire of the urinary tract: A potential paradigm shift. Journal of Clinical Microbiology. 2019;**57**(3):e00675-e00618

[14] Dubourg G, Morand A, Mekhalif F, Godefroy R, Corthier A, Yacouba A, et al. Deciphering the urinary microbiota repertoire by Culturomics reveals

mostly anaerobic bacteria from the gut. Frontiers in Microbiology. 2020;**11**:513305

[15] Thomas-White K, Forster SC, Kumar N, Van Kuiken M, Putonti C, Stares MD, et al. Culturing of female bladder bacteria reveals an interconnected urogenital microbiota. Nature Communications. 2018;**9**(1):1557

[16] Komesu YM, Richter HE, Carper B, Dinwiddie DL, Lukacz ES, Siddiqui NY, et al. The urinary microbiome in women with mixed urinary incontinence compared to similarly aged controls. International Urogynecology Journal. 2018;**29**(12):1785-1795

[17] Price TK, Hilt EE, Thomas-White K, Mueller ER, Wolfe AJ, Brubaker L. The urobiome of continent adult women: A cross-sectional study. BJOG: an International Journal of Obstetrics and Gynaecology. 2020;**127**(2):193-201

[18] Bi H, Tian Y, Song C, Li J, Liu T, Chen Z, et al. Urinary microbiota - a potential biomarker and therapeutic target for bladder cancer. Journal of Medical Microbiology. 2019;**68**(10):1471-1478

[19] Liu F, Ling Z, Xiao Y, Yang Q, Zheng L, Jiang P, et al. Characterization of the urinary microbiota of elderly women and the effects of type 2 diabetes and urinary tract infections on the microbiota. Oncotarget. 2017;**8**(59):100678-100690

[20] Liu F, Liu A, Lu X, Zhang Z, Xue Y, Xu J, et al. Dysbiosis signatures of the microbial profile in tissue from bladder cancer. Cancer Medicine. 2019;**8**(16):6904-6914

[21] Mai G, Chen L, Li R, Liu Q, Zhang H, Ma Y. Common Core bacterial biomarkers of bladder cancer based on multiple datasets. BioMed Research International. 2019;**2019**:4824909

[22] Moustafa A, Li W, Singh H, Moncera KJ, Torralba MG, Yu Y, et al. Microbial metagenome of urinary tract infection. Scientific Reports. 2018;**8**(1):4333

[23] Curtiss N, Balachandran A, Krska L, Peppiatt-Wildman C, Wildman S, Duckett J. Age, menopausal status and the bladder microbiome. European Journal of Obstetrics, Gynecology, and Reproductive Biology. 2018;**228**:126-129

[24] Paduch DA. Viral lower urinary tract infections. Current Urology Reports. 2007;**8**(4):324-335

[25] Santiago-Rodriguez TM, Ly M, Bonilla N, Pride DT. The human urine virome in association with urinary tract infections. Frontiers in Microbiology. 2015;**6**:14

[26] Garretto A, Thomas-White K, Wolfe AJ, Putonti C. Detecting viral genomes in the female urinary microbiome. The Journal of General Virology. 2018;**99**(8):1141-1146

[27] Chrisofos M, Skolarikos A, Lazaris A, Bogris S, Deliveliotis C. HPV 16/18-associated condyloma acuminatum of the urinary bladder: First international report and review of literature. International Journal of STD & AIDS. 2004;**15**(12):836-838

[28] Tshomo U, Franceschi S, Tshokey T, Tobgay T, Baussano I, Tenet V, et al. Evaluation of the performance of human papillomavirus testing in paired urine and clinician-collected cervical samples among women aged over 30 years in Bhutan. Virology Journal. 2017;**14**(1):74

[29] Iwasawa A, Kumamoto Y, Maruta H, Fukushima M, Tsukamoto T, Fujinaga K,

et al. Presence of human papillomavirus 6/11 DNA in condyloma acuminatum of the urinary bladder. Urologia Internationalis. 1992;**48**(2):235-238

[30] Karim RZ, Rose BR, Brammah S, Scolyer RA. Condylomata acuminata of the urinary bladder with HPV 11. Pathology. 2005;**37**(2):176-178

[31] Ackerman AL, Underhill DM. The mycobiome of the human urinary tract: Potential roles for fungi in urology. Annals of Translational Medicine. 2017;**5**(2):5

[32] Grine G, Lotte R, Chirio D, Chevalier A, Raoult D, Drancourt M, et al. Co-culture of Methanobrevibacter smithii with enterobacteria during urinary infection. eBioMedicine. 2019;**43**:333-337

[33] Nadler N, Kvich L, Bjarnsholt T, Jensen JB, Gögenur I, Azawi N. The discovery of bacterial biofilm in patients with muscle invasive bladder cancer. APMIS. 2021;**129**(5):265-270

[34] Saginala K, Barsouk A, Aluru JS, Rawla P, Padala SA, Barsouk A. Epidemiology of bladder cancer. Medical Sciences (Basel, Switzerland). 2020;**8**(1):15

[35] Bowa K, Mulele C, Kachimba J, Manda E, Mapulanga V, Mukosai S. A review of bladder cancer in sub-Saharan Africa: A different disease, with a distinct presentation, assessment, and treatment. Annals of African Medicine. 2018;**17**(3):99-105

[36] Inobaya MT, Olveda RM, Chau TN, Olveda DU, Ross AG. Prevention and control of schistosomiasis: A current perspective. Research and Reports in Tropical Medicine. 2014;**2014**(5):65-75

[37] Cohen SM, Ellwein LB. Cell proliferation in carcinogenesis. Science (New York, N.Y.). 1990;**249**(4972):1007-1011

[38] Mostafa MH, Helmi S, Badawi AF, Tricker AR, Spiegelhalder B, Preussmann R. Nitrate, nitrite and volatile N-nitroso compounds in the urine of Schistosoma haematobium and Schistosoma mansoni infected patients. Carcinogenesis. 1994;**15**(4):619-625

[39] Johansson SL, Cohen SM. Epidemiology and etiology of bladder cancer. Seminars in Surgical Oncology. 1997;**13**(5):291-298

[40] Adebayo AS, Suryavanshi MV, Bhute S, Agunloye AM, Isokpehi RD, Anumudu CI, et al. The microbiome in urogenital schistosomiasis and induced bladder pathologies. PLoS Neglected Tropical Diseases. 2017;**11**(8):e0005826

[41] Yacouba A, Tidjani Alou M, Lagier J-C, Dubourg G, Raoult D. Urinary microbiota and bladder cancer: A systematic review and a focus on uropathogens. Seminars in Cancer Biology. 2022. DOI: 10.1016/j.semcancer.2021.12.010

[42] Wu P, Zhang G, Zhao J, Chen J, Chen Y, Huang W, et al. Profiling the urinary microbiota in male patients with bladder cancer in China. Frontiers in Cellular and Infection Microbiology. 2018;**8**:167

[43] Bučević Popović V, Šitum M, Chow CT, Chan LS, Roje B, Terzić J. The urinary microbiome associated with bladder cancer. Scientific Reports. 2018;**8**(1):12157

[44] McConnell MJ, Actis L, Pachón J. Acinetobacter baumannii: Human infections, factors contributing to pathogenesis and animal models. FEMS Microbiology Reviews. 2013;**37**(2):130-155

[45] Roperto S, Di Guardo G, Leonardi L, Pagnini U, Manco E, Paciello O, et al.

Bacterial isolates from the urine of cattle affected by urothelial tumors of the urinary bladder. Research in Veterinary Science. 2012;**93**(3):1361-1366

[46] Lotte R, Lotte L, Ruimy R. Actinotignum schaalii (formerly Actinobaculum schaalii): A newly recognized pathogen-review of the literature. Clinical Microbiology and Infection. 2016;**22**(1):28-36

[47] Xu W, Yang L, Lee P, Huang WC, Nossa C, Ma Y, et al. Mini-review: Perspective of the microbiome in the pathogenesis of urothelial carcinoma. American Journal of Clinical and Experimental Urology. 2014;**2**(1):57-61

[48] Alfano M, Canducci F, Nebuloni M, Clementi M, Montorsi F, Salonia A. The interplay of extracellular matrix and microbiome in urothelial bladder cancer. Nature Reviews Urology. 2016;**13**(2):77-90

[49] Goldufsky J, Wood S, Hajihossainlou B, Rehman T, Majdobeh O, Kaufman HL, et al. Pseudomonas aeruginosa exotoxin T induces potent cytotoxicity against a variety of murine and human cancer cell lines. Journal of Medical Microbiology. 2015;**64**(Pt 2):164-173

[50] Pederzoli F, Ferrarese R, Amato V, Locatelli I, Alchera E, Lucianò R, et al. Sex-specific alterations in the urinary and tissue microbiome in therapy-naïve urothelial bladder cancer patients. European Urology Oncology. 2020;**3**(6):784-788

[51] Vétizou M, Pitt JM, Daillère R, Lepage P, Waldschmitt N, Flament C, et al. Anticancer immunotherapy by CTLA-4 blockade relies on the gut microbiota. Science. 2015;**350**(6264):1079-1084

[52] Kertesz MA, Kawasaki A. Hydrocarbon-degrading Sphingomonads: Sphingomonas, Sphingobium, Novosphingobium, and Sphingopyxis. In: Timmis KN, editor. Handbook of Hydrocarbon and Lipid Microbiology. Berlin, Heidelberg: Springer Berlin Heidelberg; 2010. pp. 1693-1705

[53] Moynihan M, Sullivan T, Provenzano K, Rieger-Christ K. Urinary microbiome evaluation in patients presenting with hematuria with a focus on exposure to tobacco smoke. Research and Reports in Urology. 2019;**11**:359-367

[54] Oresta B, Braga D, Lazzeri M, Frego N, Saita A, Faccani C, et al. The microbiome of catheter collected urine in males with bladder cancer according to disease stage. Journal of Urology. 2021;**205**(1):86-93

[55] Chen YE, Fischbach MA, Belkaid Y. Skin microbiota–host interactions. Nature. 2018;**553**(7689):427-436

[56] Hussein AA, Elsayed AS, Durrani M, Jing Z, Iqbal U, Gomez EC, et al. Investigating the association between the urinary microbiome and bladder cancer: An exploratory study. Urologic Oncology: Seminars and Original Investigations. 2021;**39**(6):370.e9-370e19

[57] Mansour B, Monyók Á, Makra N, Gajdács M, Vadnay I, Ligeti B, et al. Bladder cancer-related microbiota: Examining differences in urine and tissue samples. Scientific Reports. 2020;**10**(1):11042

[58] Wilson MR, Jiang Y, Villalta PW, Stornetta A, Boudreau PD, Carrá A, et al. The human gut bacterial genotoxin colibactin alkylates. DNA. 2019;**363**(6428):eaar7785

[59] Hill C, Guarner F, Reid G, Gibson GR, Merenstein DJ, Pot B, et al. Expert consensus document. The

international scientific Association for Probiotics and Prebiotics consensus statement on the scope and appropriate use of the term probiotic. Nature Reviews Gastroenterology & Hepatology. 2014;**11**(8):506-514

[60] Kim J-M, Park Y-J. Lactobacillus and urine microbiome in association with urinary tract infections and bacterial vaginosis. UTI. 2018;**13**(1):7-13

[61] Jiang L, Xiao X, Ren J, Tang Y, Weng H, Yang Q, et al. Proteomic analysis of bladder cancer indicates Prx-I as a key molecule in BI-TK/GCV treatment system. PLoS One. 2014;**9**(6):e98764

[62] Myles IA, Castillo CR, Barbian KD, Kanakabandi K, Virtaneva K, Fitzmeyer E, et al. Therapeutic responses to Roseomonas mucosa in atopic dermatitis may involve lipid-mediated TNF-related epithelial repair. Science Translational Medicine. 2020;**12**(560):eaaz8631

[63] Wicaksono DP, Washio J, Abiko Y, Domon H, Takahashi N. Nitrite production from nitrate and its link with lactate metabolism in Oral Veillonella spp. Applied and Environmental Microbiology. 2020;**86**(20):e01255-e01220

[64] Barry KH, Jones RR, Cantor KP, Beane Freeman LE, Wheeler DC, Baris D, et al. Ingested nitrate and nitrite and bladder cancer in northern New England. Epidemiology (Cambridge, Mass). 2020;**31**(1):136-144

[65] Marzhoseyni Z, Shojaie L, Tabatabaei SA, Movahedpour A, Safari M, Esmaeili D, et al. Streptococcal bacterial components in cancer therapy. Cancer Gene Therapy. 2022;**29**(2):141-155

[66] Mager DL. Bacteria and cancer: Cause, coincidence or cure? A review. Journal of Translational Medicine. 2006;**4**(1):14

[67] Ohashi Y, Nakai S, Tsukamoto T, Masumori N, Akaza H, Miyanaga N, et al. Habitual intake of lactic acid bacteria and risk reduction of bladder cancer. Urologia Internationalis. 2002;**68**(4):273-280

[68] Larsson SC, Andersson SO, Johansson JE, Wolk A. Cultured milk, yogurt, and dairy intake in relation to bladder cancer risk in a prospective study of Swedish women and men. The American Journal of Clinical Nutrition. 2008;**88**(4):1083-1087

[69] Aso Y, Akazan H, BLP Study Group. Prophylactic effect of a lactobacillus casei preparation on the recurrence of superficial bladder cancer. Urologia Internationalis. 1992;**49**(3):125-129

[70] Feyisetan O, Tracey C, Hellawell GO. Probiotics, dendritic cells and bladder cancer. BJU International. 2012;**109**(11):1594-1597

[71] Naito S, Koga H, Yamaguchi A, Fujimoto N, Hasui Y, Kuramoto H, et al. Prevention of recurrence with epirubicin and lactobacillus casei after transurethral resection of bladder cancer. The Journal of Urology. 2008;**179**(2):485-490

[72] Zasloff M. Antimicrobial peptides, innate immunity, and the normally sterile urinary tract. Journal of the American Society of Nephrology. 2007;**18**(11):2810

[73] McMillan A, Macklaim JM, Burton JP, Reid G. Adhesion of lactobacillus iners AB-1 to human fibronectin: A key mediator for persistence in the vagina? Reproductive Sciences (Thousand Oaks, Calif). 2013;**20**(7):791-796

[74] Hopkins AM, Kichenadasse G, Karapetis CS, Rowland A, Sorich MJ.

Concomitant antibiotic use and survival in urothelial carcinoma treated with Atezolizumab. European Urology. 2020;**78**(4):540-543

[75] Pederzoli F, Bandini M, Raggi D, Marandino L, Basile G, Alfano M, et al. Is there a detrimental effect of antibiotic therapy in patients with muscle-invasive bladder cancer treated with Neoadjuvant Pembrolizumab? European Urology. 2021;**80**(3):319-322

Chapter 3

Intracorporeal Urinary Diversion of Robot-Assisted Radical Cystectomy

Yasukazu Nakanishi, Shugo Yajima and Hitoshi Masuda

Abstract

With the widespread utilization of robot-assisted radical cystectomy (RARC) that demonstrated non-inferiority compared to open radical cystectomy in terms of several outcomes, urinary diversions are now performed for both extracorporeal and intracorporeal procedures. The potential benefits of intracorporeal urinary diversion (ICUD) include smaller incisions, reduced pain, reduced intraoperative blood loss, reduced bowel handling and exposure, and third space loss. ICUD following radical cystectomy requires many steps and a careful stepwise progression. Surgical volumes (RARCs per year) per center and per surgeon appear to be correlated with a reduction in complications. The European Association of Urology guidelines recommend that hospitals should perform at least 10, and preferably more than 20 operations annually. With the aim of generalizing ICUD, this chapter will discuss the following items: (1) Technique of intracorporeal ileal conduit; (2) Perioperative comparison of intracorporeal and extracorporeal urinary diversion in RARC; (3) Hybrid technique in robot-assisted intracorporeal ileal conduit; and (4) Intracorporeal ileal neobladder.

Keywords: intracorporeal urinary diversion, robot-assisted radical cystectomy, ileal conduit, ileal neobladder, surgical technique, perioperative outcomes

1. Introduction

Over the last decade, robot-assisted radical cystectomy (RARC) has been gradually adopted and has been shown to maintain oncological equivalence compared to open radical cystectomy (ORC) [1–4], including in randomized control trials (RCTs) [5–10]. In addition, RCT evaluating quality of life have reported stability in RARC compared to ORC [11]. The development of minimally invasive surgical techniques has been widely used in a variety of surgical with the adaptation of minimally invasive techniques is to minimize surgical morbidity and improve recovery. With regard to urinary diversion following radical cystectomy, intracorporeal urinary diversion (ICUD) has become more common in recent years in place of extracorporeal urinary diversion (ECUD). According to data of the International Robotic Cystectomy Consortium (IRCC) database, comprising data from 26 institutions, ICUD increased at a rate of 9–11% per year, from 9% of all urinary diversions in 2005 to 97% in 2015 [12]. This trend was also observed for intracorporeal ileal neobladder alone [13]. This chapter mainly explains ICUD techniques and perioperative outcomes.

2. Technique of intracorporeal ileal conduit

This chapter describes the method when using the da Vinci Surgical System (Intuitive Surgical Inc., Sunnyvale, CA, USA).

2.1 Port placement

Port placement is similar to robot-assisted radical prostatectomy (RARP), and both assistant ports are often 12 mm ports. All ports are placed approximately 2 cm higher than the usual position for RARP.

2.2 Preliminary steps of ICUD

After the completion of radical cystectomy, specimens are placed in an impermeable retrieval bag. In female patients, the specimen may be extracted through the vagina. In male patients, the specimens can be removed either through the subsequent ostomy sites or by enlarging the 12-mm camera port. Before undocking, the left ureter is guided to the right side through the back of the sigmoid colon and fixed to the ventral peritoneum through support threads over both ureters.

2.3 Repositioning

The robot is undocked and the Trendelenburg position is returned to 0–15 degrees. The robot is then re-docked in this new bed position. This maneuver allows the small bowel to return to the lower abdomen and pelvis, facilitating subsequent bowel manipulation for the intracorporeal diversion.

2.4 Determination of the ileal segment for diversion

The first step is to identify the ileocecal junction. Preserve at least 20 cm of ileum proximal to the ileocecal valve by introducing a 20-cm silk suture into the abdomen and using it to measure the length and distance of the bowel tract (**Figure 1A**). A segment of ileum is then identified and selected for the urinary diversion, tagging the proximal and distal ends of the bowel (**Figure 1B**). A 15–20 cm length of ileum is then resected depending on the patient's body habitus. Cadiere forceps, which are less traumatic than the Prograsp or Maryland forceps, are recommended for bowel manipulation.

2.5 Ileal resection and reconstruction

After creating two mesenteric windows, the bowel lumen is divided proximally and distally by introducing a 45 or 60 mm stapler into the lateral assistant port using the da Vinci Xi Endo Wrist Stapler with SmartClamp technology. Indocyanine green (ICG) and the Firefly system may be used when undergoing ileal resection [14]. Proximal and distal bowel ends are identified and positioned in a side-to-side fashion. After the closed end of the bowel has been cut off with scissors and released, the da Vinci Xi Endo Wrist Stapler is inserted in the bowel segment, and side to side bowel anastomosis is carried out using one 45 or 60 mm bowel loads (**Figure 1C**). A final 45 or 60 mm bowel load closes the horizontal part. The mesenteric window is closed with a shallow running suture to prevent internal bowel herniation.

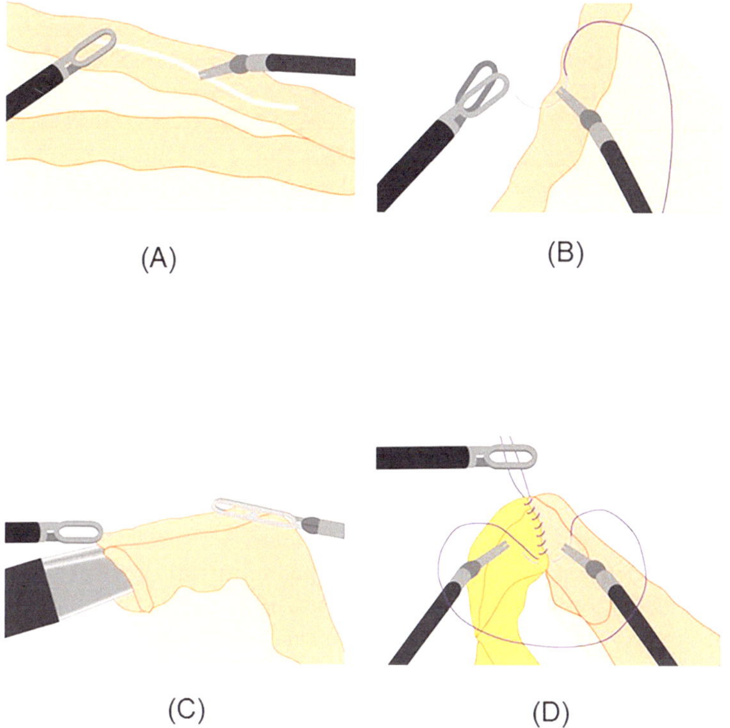

Figure 1.
(A) Measuring distance of terminal ileum; (B) tagging the ileum to mark the incision site; (C) the stapler is closed and fired to create the anastomosis; (D) creation of Wallace posterior plate.

2.6 Ileal conduit diversion

Here we describe the Wallace surgical technique for uretero-ileal anastomosis [15]. The first step is to create the uretero-uretero anastomosis. The distal end of both ureters are spatulated using Monopolar Scissors to at least 20 mm to match the caliber of the ileum. The distal end of both spatulated ureters are marked as stay sutures using a 4/0 absorbable suture. The inner opposite borders of both ureters are over-sewn using a running fashion with a 4/0 absorbable suture. The uretero-ileal anastomosis is constructed with two 15 cm lengths of 4/0 absorbable suture in a running fashion from the heel of the spatulation to the toe on each side (**Figure 1D**). After ureteroileal anastomosis is completed, a 6-Fr single-J ureteral stents are inserted into each ureter. A robotic arm is passed through the ileal conduit to guide the stent outside the ureter to the distal side of the ileal conduit. Then the anterior side of urtero-ileal anastomosis is completed. The right robotic arm is undocked and the assistant makes the stoma in the standard fashion.

3. Perioperative comparison of intracorporeal and extracorporeal urinary diversion in RARC

To date, although several observational studies have suggested advantages of ICUD over EUCD, there are no RCTs comparing the differences between these two operative methods.

The systematic review and meta-analysis [16] evaluating the perioperative outcomes between ICUD and ECUD reported no significant differences in overall and major complications between ICUD and ECUD. A subgroup analysis of high-volume centers showed that ICUD was significantly associated with a reduced risk of major complications [OR 0.57, 95% confidence interval (CI) 0.37–0.86, $p = 0.008$]. In terms of perioperative outcomes, estimated blood loss (EBL) and blood transfusion rates were significantly lower in patients who underwent an ICUD compared to those who underwent ECUD. In contrast, operative time, length of stay (LOS), and ileus and gastrointestinal (GI) related complications were not significantly different between these two methods. A subgroup analysis of low-volume centers showed that EBL and blood transfusion rates were significantly lower in patients who underwent ICUD (mean difference −121.6 ml, 95% CI −160.9 to −82.3, $p < 0.00001$ and OR 0.36, 95% CI 0.20–0.62, $p = 0.00003$, respectively).

Another systematic review and meta-analysis [17] reported that ICUD and ECUD had comparable early (<30 days) and late (30–90 days) complication rates. In terms of perioperative outcomes, EBL tended to be lower in patients who underwent an ICUD compared to those who underwent ECUD (mean difference –86 ml, 95% CI −124 to –48, $p = 0.058$). The transfusion rate was significantly lower in the ICUD group, 4.6% versus 13.9% in the ECUD group ($p < 0.001$). The weighed mean difference of operative time in the ICUD and ECUD group was 16 (95% CI −34 to 66).

There is a caveat to these studies' results. A relatively large number of urologists choose ECUD in the early stages of RARC implementation and then introduce ICUDs when they are proficient. Thus the results should be compared between the final period of ECUD and the period of ICUD implementation. With respect to proficiency after the introduction of ICUD, approximately 30 cases are expected to be needed to stabilize perioperative outcomes. In the Learning Curve estimate for RARC, almost 30 cases have been agreed upon for this particular procedure to achieve a lymph node yield of 20 and a positive resection margin rate of 5% or less [18]. A study that evaluated learning curves for three groups of approximately 30 cases each of 100 patients initially introduced to RARC revealed that the transfusion rate was low and stable after approximately 30 cases [19]. On the other hand, a retrospective analysis at a high-volume hospital reported that more than 137 cases were needed to stabilize perioperative outcomes, including major complications in 90 days, highlighting the need for substantial experience [20].

According to the systematic review and meta-analysis by Tanneru et al. [17], ICUD ileal conduits are more likely to be performed, especially in hospitals with more than 100 cases [12, 21, 22]. This is presumably because neobladder formation may be technically difficult and patient selection is more rigorous than with ileal conduits.

It has been noted that the ECUD group tends to have higher transfusion rates than the ICUD group. Several studies have shown that blood transfusions are associated with an increased risk of cancer recurrence and mortality after radical cystectomy, indicating the importance of reduced transfusion rates for oncologic outcomes [23, 24]. For intracorporeal ileal neobladder alone, analysis of a retrospective review of IRCC database reported that patients who underwent intracorporeal ileal neobladder had shorter hospital stays and fewer 30 day reoperations but were readmitted more frequently compared to those who underwent extracorporeal ileal neobladder [13].

While there is reportedly no difference in overall complication rates, ECUD is associated with a higher incidence of GI complications. It has been suggested that the reason for this is related to the fact that open surgery exposes the peritoneum to air, which is associated with an inflammatory response and can lead to postoperative ileus [25, 26]. According to IRCC analysis, GI complications were significantly higher in patients who received ECUD (23%) compared to the patients who received ICUD (10%) [1]. With regard to the incidence of Grade 3 or higher GI, complications were reported to be significantly higher in ECUD group than ICUD group [27]. However, a study comparing 972 patients found no difference between these two methods [12]. From another viewpoint, since early mobilization and low Geriatric-8, etc. have been identified as causes of postoperative ileus development, such attention may be warranted [28].

Another typical complication of urinary diversion is ureteroenteric strictures. When anastomotic stricture occurs, surgical intervention, including invasive anastomotic reshaping, is often required. The up to 13% incidence of ureteroenteric stricture has been reported, depending on the definition, and includes both ICUD and ECUD [29]. According to the study, which evaluated the stricture rate in intracorporeal diversions with and without the use of ICG for perfusion evaluation of the distal ureter [30], stricture formation was 0% in the ICG group compared to 10.6% per patient in the non-ICG group at 12 months follow up. In an evaluation using ICG with SPY fluorescence at ECUD, the stricture rate was 0% in the ICG group versus 7.5% in the non-ICG group. The median length excised for ureters with poor distal perfusion was 3.8 cm, compared with 2.2 cm for ureters with good distal perfusion [31]. A retrospective study evaluating both methods in 127 patients reported a 3.2% incidence of stricture for ICUD and 7.4% for ECUD, with no difference between these 2 groups [22].

4. Hybrid technique in robot-assisted intracorporeal ileal conduit

The advantages of ICUD are smaller incisions, less pain, and less bowel exposure compared to ECUD [32–34]. ICUD tends to have a longer operative time in the early stages of implementation due to the complexity of the technique and steep learning curve [18, 19, 35]. The implementation of new surgical techniques requires careful stepwise progression in order to protect patients as much as possible against potential harms associated with such implementation. Herein, we describe a hybrid ICUD procedure that partially incorporates ECUD techniques.

4.1 Preliminary steps

After the completion of radical cystectomy and pelvic lymphadenectomy, the left ureter is moved to the right side of the abdomen through a window created in the mesentery behind the sigmoid colon. The robot is undocked and the Trendelenburg position is returned to 0–15 degrees.

4.2 Extracorporeal part

An extended incision (approximately 4–6 cm) is made through the camera port and the specimen is removed from the body. The incision is then covered with Smart Retractor® (TOP Inc., Tokyo, Japan). Isolate an ileal segment (approximately 15–20 cm) at least 20 cm from the ileocecal valve (**Figure 2A**). The lumen of the isolated ileum (conduit) is cleaned with saline. A skin incision is made at the site of stoma creation, creating a stoma hole. The distal end of the conduit is then pulled out of the abdominal wall through the stoma hole. Approximately 20 cm length of silk thread is ligated at the distal end of the conduit and used as a support thread (**Figure 2B**). The collected ileum is then returned to the abdominal cavity, and the wound at the stoma site is temporarily closed with silk suture. The Smart Retractor® is covered with Free Access® (TOP Inc, Tokyo, Japan), and the abdominal cavity is re-insufflated (**Figure 2C**).

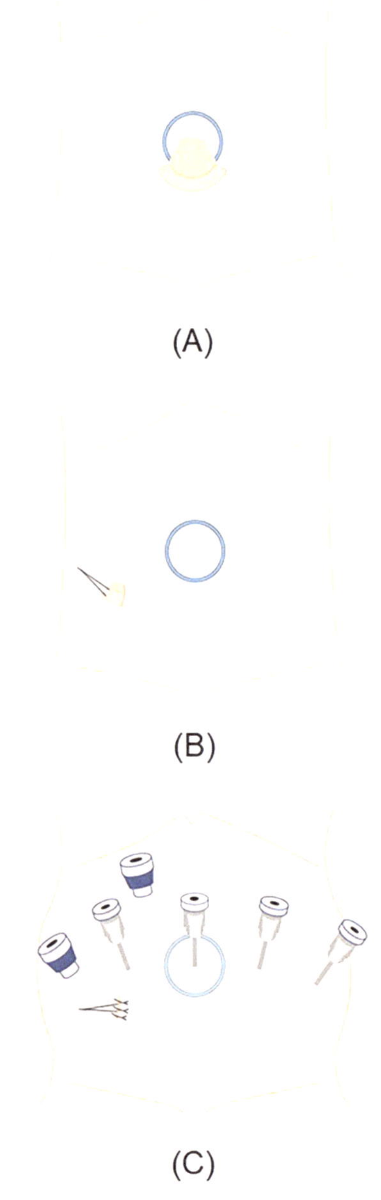

Figure 2.
(A) Extended wound and ileum harvested (approximately 20 cm); (B) Ileum temporarily pulled out through the abdominal wall and ligated with silk threads; (C) return the conduit to the abdominal cavity and re-insufflate.

4.3 Intracorporeal part

The robot is then re-docked to perform uretero-ileal anastomosis intracorporeally. Uretero-ileal anastomosis is performed by the Wallace method described above.

This method is useful until the surgeon becomes accustomed to intracorporeal manipulation.

5. Intracorporeal ileal neobladder

Bowel handling in ICUD is often a limiting step in surgical learning. Intracorporeal ileal neobladder in particular requires attention because of its large number of intraoperative manipulations. A tertiary reference center reported that 60 cases are required to stabilize the perioperative outcomes [36].

Several intracorporeal neobladder techniques were recently reported, including Studer "U" [37–42], Hautmann "W" [43], "Y" pouch [44, 45], Pyramid pouch [46], Padua style [47], Vesicia ileale Padovana [48], FloRIN style [49] with promising perioperative outcomes.

We describe a J-shaped orthotopic neobladder based on the Studer method. This procedure is relatively simple to perform.

5.1 Determination of the ileal segment for diversion

A 50 cm portion is selected, leaving at least 20 cm of ileum proximal to the ileocecal valve, and including the portion of the ileum closest to the pelvic floor. Ileal resection and reconstruction are performed as described above.

5.2 Detubularization and reshaping the ileum into a spherical neobladder

Approximately 40 cm of antimesenteric border of distal ileum is opened whereas the proximal 10 cm is maintained for afferent limb (**Figure 3A**). A 40 cm portion of the ileum is folded in two, and the posterior plate is then reconstructed using a 3/0 absorbable suture in a running fashion (**Figure 3B**). Single–J stents are placed over guide wire and the ends are advanced through the wall of the afferent limb (**Figure 3C**). The neobladder is then symmetrically folded into a spherical reservoir applying the same suture (**Figure 3D**). An opening is then made at the most dependent portion and a urethra-ileal anastomosis is performed by using a 3/0 "barbed" running suture, starting at 5 o'clock on the urethra and then proceeding clockwise. A 20 French Foley catheter is introduced into the neobladder.

5.3 Uretero-enteral anastomosis and stent placement

The anastomosis between the ureters and the afferent limb is performed using the Wallace technique. Both ureters are then anastomosed to the afferent limb using a 4/0 absorbable suture in a running fashion. The caudal side of stents are advanced to the abdominal wall through the 5 mm trocar, and then stents are pushed up through ureters to renal pelvis. The remaining part of Wallace plate is closed (**Figure 3E**) and its water–tightness is tested accordingly.

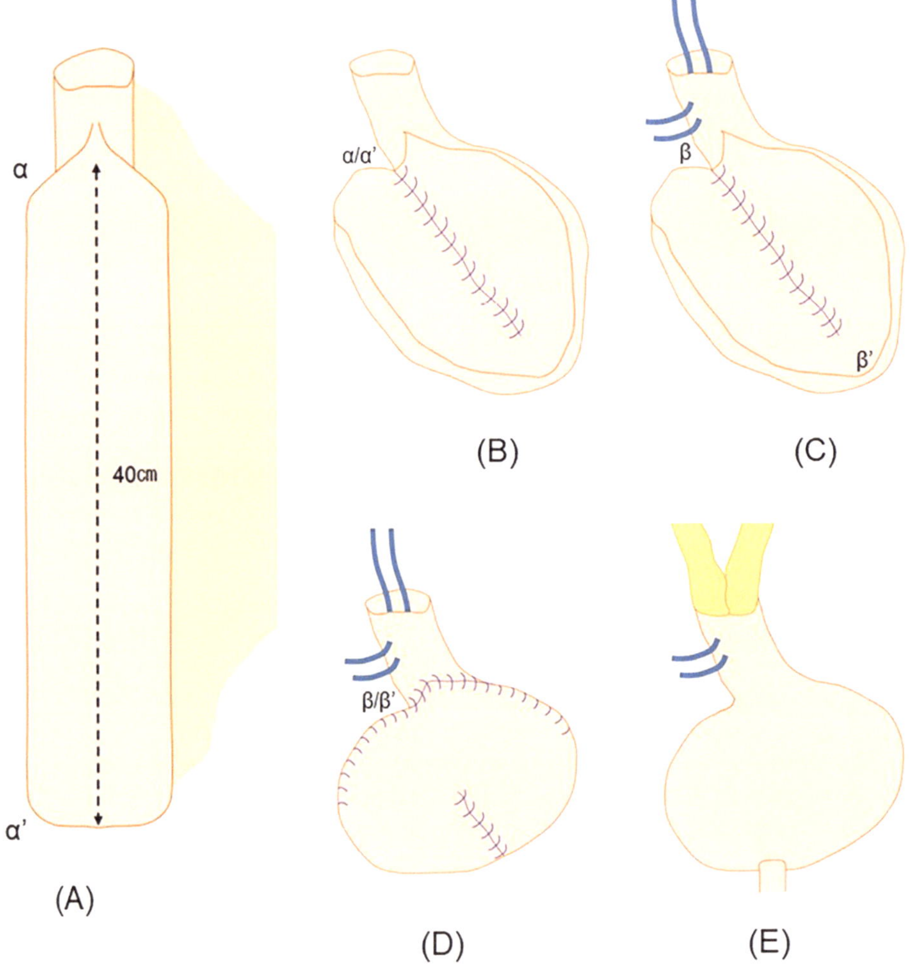

Figure 3.
(A) Detublarized ileum; (B) posterior plate of ileal neobladder (α overlaps with α'); (C) situation with ureteral stents through the afferent limb; (D) spherical reshaped reservoir (β overlaps with β'); (E) situation after completion of urinary tract anastomosis.

5.4 Postoperative management

Manual irrigation of the neobladder is performed intermittently every 8 hours. It should be noted that mucus volume will be increased after resumption of eating. The drain is removed when the amount of fluid is <200 ml. The ureteral stents are removed on the seventh postoperative day under urethrocystography. The urethral catheter is removed 3–4 weeks after operation.

5.5 Functional outcome

Functional outcomes are related to many factors such as age, mental or cognitive status, reservoir volume, and urethral length. The day time urinary continence recovery rates with less than one pad per day performed by intracorporeal Studer's method were reported to be 62–88% at 1 year [50, 51]. A study including only a small number of 12 men reported a 100% day time urinary abstinence recovery rate defined as <1 pad per day at 1 year [52]. Retrospective study compared continence rates of RARC with intracorporeal and extracorporeal orthotopic neobladders revealed that no statistically significant difference was found in continence recovery rates [53]. In terms of potency, the recovery rate was 81.2% in nerve-sparing patients with or without PDE5 medication at 1 year (with PDE5: 50% or without medication: 31.2%, respectively) [50].

6. Conclusions

Complications of RARC with ICUD in the short-term and midterm periods were equivalent to those of ECUD. In high volume centers, ICUD tends to have fewer major complications. Furthermore, ICUD tends to have a lower incidence of GI complications than ECUD, suggesting that ICUD may be a preferred method for urinary diversion.

Conflict of interest

The authors declare no conflict of interest.

Author details

Yasukazu Nakanishi*, Shugo Yajima and Hitoshi Masuda
Department of Urology, National Cancer Center Hospital East, Kashiwa, Chiba, Japan

*Address all correspondence to: yanakani@east.ncc.go.jp

References

[1] Ahmed K, Khan SA, Hayn MH, Agarwal PK, Badani KK, Balbay MD, et al. Analysis of intracorporeal compared with extracorporeal urinary diversion after robot-assisted radical cystectomy: Results from the International Robotic Cystectomy Consortium. European Urology. 2014;**65**(2):340-347

[2] Novara G, Catto JW, Wilson T, Annerstedt M, Chan K, Murphy DG, et al. Systematic review and cumulative analysis of perioperative outcomes and complications after robot-assisted radical cystectomy. European Urology. 2015;**67**(3):376-401

[3] Leow JJ, Reese SW, Jiang W, Lipsitz SR, Bellmunt J, Trinh QD, et al. Propensity-matched comparison of morbidity and costs of open and robot-assisted radical cystectomies: a contemporary population-based analysis in the United States. European Urology. 2014;**66**(3):569-576

[4] Hu JC, Chughtai B, O'Malley P, Halpern JA, Mao J, Scherr DS, et al. Perioperative outcomes, health care costs, and survival after robotic-assisted versus open radical cystectomy: a National Comparative Effectiveness Study. European Urology. 2016;**70**(1):195-202

[5] Parekh DJ, Reis IM, Castle EP, Gonzalgo ML, Woods ME, Svatek RS, et al. Robot-assisted radical cystectomy versus open radical cystectomy in patients with bladder cancer (RAZOR): an open-label, randomised, phase 3, non-inferiority trial. The Lancet. 2018;**391**(10139):2525-2536

[6] Bochner BH, Dalbagni G, Marzouk KH, Sjoberg DD, Lee J, Donat SM, et al. Randomized trial comparing open radical cystectomy and robot-assisted laparoscopic radical cystectomy: oncologic outcomes. European Urology. 2018;**74**(4): 465-471

[7] Khan MS, Gan C, Ahmed K, Ismail AF, Watkins J, Summers JA, et al. A single-centre early phase randomised controlled three-arm trial of open, robotic, and laparoscopic radical cystectomy (CORAL). European Urology. 2016;**69**(4):613-621

[8] Catto JWF, Khetrapal P, Ricciardi F, Ambler G, Williams NR, Al-Hammouri T, et al. Effect of robot-assisted radical cystectomy with intracorporeal urinary diversion vs open radical cystectomy on 90-day morbidity and mortality among patients with bladder cancer: a randomized clinical trial. Journal of the American Medical Association. 2022

[9] Mastroianni R, Ferriero M, Tuderti G, Anceschi U, Bove AM, Brassetti A, et al. Open radical cystectomy versus robot-assisted radical cystectomy with intracorporeal urinary diversion: early outcomes of a single-center randomized controlled trial. The Journal of Urology. 2022;**207**(5):982-992

[10] Maibom SL, Roder MA, Aasvang EK, Rohrsted M, Thind PO, Bagi P, et al. Open vs robot-assisted radical cystectomy (BORARC): a double-blinded, randomised feasibility study. BJU International. 2021;**130**(1):102-113

[11] Vejlgaard M, Maibom SL, Joensen UN, Thind PO, Rohrsted M, Aasvang EK, et al. Quality of life and secondary outcomes for open versus robot-assisted radical cystectomy: a

double-blinded, randomised feasibility trial. World Journal of Urology. 2022;**40**(7):1669-1677

[12] Hussein AA, May PR, Jing Z, Ahmed YE, Wijburg CJ, Canda AE, et al. Outcomes of intracorporeal urinary diversion after robot-assisted radical cystectomy: results from the International Robotic Cystectomy Consortium. The Journal of Urology. 2018;**199**(5):1302-1311

[13] Dalimov Z, Iqbal U, Jing Z, Wiklund P, Kaouk J, Kim E, et al. Intracorporeal versus extracorporeal neobladder after robot-assisted radical cystectomy: results from the International Robotic Cystectomy Consortium. Urology. 2022;**159**:127-132

[14] Jeglinschi S, Carlier M, Denimal L, Guillonneau B, Chevallier D, Tibi B, et al. Intracorporeal urinary diversion during robot-assisted radical cystectomy using indocyanine green. The Canadian Journal of Urology. 2020;**27**(5):10394-10401

[15] Wallace DM. Ureteric diversion using a conduit: a simplified technique. British Journal of Urology. 1966;**38**(5):522-527

[16] Katayama S, Mori K, Pradere B, Mostafaei H, Schuettfort VM, Quhal F, et al. Intracorporeal versus extracorporeal urinary diversion in robot-assisted radical cystectomy: a systematic review and meta-analysis. International Journal of Clinical Oncology. 2021;**26**(9):1587-1599

[17] Tanneru K, Jazayeri SB, Kumar J, Alam MU, Norez D, Nguyen S, et al. Intracorporeal versus extracorporeal urinary diversion following robot-assisted radical cystectomy: a meta-analysis, cumulative analysis, and systematic review. Journal of Robotic Surgery. 2021;**15**(3):321-333

[18] Hayn MH, Hussain A, Mansour AM, Andrews PE, Carpentier P, Castle E, et al. The learning curve of robot-assisted radical cystectomy: results from the International Robotic Cystectomy Consortium. European Urology. 2010;**58**(2):197-202

[19] Porreca A, Mineo Bianchi F, Romagnoli D, D'Agostino D, Corsi P, Giampaoli M, et al. Robot-assisted radical cystectomy with totally intracorporeal urinary diversion: surgical and early functional outcomes through the learning curve in a single high-volume center. Journal of Robotic Surgery. 2020;**14**(2):261-269

[20] Wijburg CJ, Hannink G, Michels CTJ, Weijerman PC, Issa R, Tay A, et al. Learning curve analysis for intracorporeal robot-assisted radical cystectomy: results from the EAU Robotic Urology Section Scientific Working Group. European Urology Open Science. 2022;**39**:55-61

[21] Lenfant L, Verhoest G, Campi R, Parra J, Graffeille V, Masson-Lecomte A, et al. Perioperative outcomes and complications of intracorporeal vs extracorporeal urinary diversion after robot-assisted radical cystectomy for bladder cancer: a real-life, multi-institutional french study. World Journal of Urology. 2018;**36**(11):1711-1718

[22] Tan TW, Nair R, Saad S, Thurairaja R, Khan MS. Safe transition from extracorporeal to intracorporeal urinary diversion following robot-assisted cystectomy: a recipe for reducing operative time, blood loss and complication rates. World Journal of Urology. 2019;**37**(2):367-372

[23] Gierth M, Aziz A, Fritsche HM, Burger M, Otto W, Zeman F, et al. The effect of intra- and postoperative allogenic blood transfusion on

patients' survival undergoing radical cystectomy for urothelial carcinoma of the bladder. World Journal of Urology. 2014;**32**(6):1447-1453

[24] Linder BJ, Frank I, Cheville JC, Tollefson MK, Thompson RH, Tarrell RF, et al. The impact of perioperative blood transfusion on cancer recurrence and survival following radical cystectomy. European Urology. 2013;**63**(5):839-845

[25] Zhang JH, Ericson KJ, Thomas LJ, Knorr J, Khanna A, Crane A, et al. Large single institution comparison of perioperative outcomes and complications of open radical cystectomy, intracorporeal robot-assisted radical cystectomy and robotic extracorporeal approach. The Journal of Urology. 2020;**203**(3):512-521

[26] Bertolo R, Agudelo J, Garisto J, Armanyous S, Fergany A, Kaouk J. Perioperative outcomes and complications after robotic radical cystectomy with intracorporeal or extracorporeal ileal conduit urinary diversion: head-to-head comparison from a single-institutional prospective study. Urology. 2019;**129**:98-105

[27] Shim JS, Kwon TG, Rha KH, Lee YG, Lee JY, Jeong BC, et al. Do patients benefit from total intracorporeal robotic radical cystectomy?: a comparative analysis with extracorporeal robotic radical cystectomy from a Korean multicenter study. Investigative and Clinical Urology. 2020;**61**(1):11-18

[28] Zennami K, Sumitomo M, Hasegawa K, Kozako M, Takahara K, Nukaya T, et al. Risk factors for postoperative ileus after robot-assisted radical cystectomy with intracorporeal urinary diversion. International Journal of Urology. 2022;**29**(6):553-558

[29] Ericson KJ, Thomas LJ, Zhang JH, Knorr JM, Khanna A, Crane A, et al. Uretero-enteric anastomotic stricture following radical cystectomy: a comparison of open, robotic extracorporeal, and robotic intracorporeal approaches. Urology. 2020;**144**:130-135

[30] Ahmadi N, Ashrafi AN, Hartman N, Shakir A, Cacciamani GE, Freitas D, et al. Use of indocyanine green to minimise uretero-enteric strictures after robotic radical cystectomy. BJU International. 2019;**124**(2):302-307

[31] Shen JK, Jamnagerwalla J, Yuh BE, Bassett MR, Chenam A, Warner JN, et al. Real-time indocyanine green angiography with the SPY fluorescence imaging platform decreases benign ureteroenteric strictures in urinary diversions performed during radical cystectomy. Therapeutic Advances in Urology. 2019;**11**:1756287219839631

[32] Presicce F, Leonardo C, Tuderti G, Brassetti A, Mastroianni R, Bove A, et al. Late complications of robot-assisted radical cystectomy with totally intracorporeal urinary diversion. World Journal of Urology. 2021;**39**(6):1903-1909

[33] Patel HR, Santos PB, de Oliveira MC, Muller S. Is robotic-assisted radical cystectomy (RARC) with intracorporeal diversion becoming the new gold standard of care? World Journal of Urology. 2016;**34**(1):25-32

[34] Dason S, Goh AC. Contemporary techniques and outcomes of robotic cystectomy and intracorporeal urinary diversions. Current Opinion in Urology. 2018;**28**(2):115-122

[35] Collins JW, Tyritzis S, Nyberg T, Schumacher MC, Laurin O, Adding C, et al. Robot-assisted radical cystectomy (RARC) with intracorporeal neobladder -

what is the effect of the learning curve on outcomes? BJU International. 2014;**113**(1):100-107

[36] LombardoR,MastroianniR,TudertiG, Ferriero M, Brassetti A, Anceschi U, et al. Benchmarking PASADENA consensus along the learning curve of robotic radical cystectomy with intracorporeal neobladder: CUSUM based assessment. Journal of Clinical Medicine. 2021;**10**(24):5969

[37] Jonsson MN, Adding LC, Hosseini A, Schumacher MC, Volz D, Nilsson A, et al. Robot-assisted radical cystectomy with intracorporeal urinary diversion in patients with transitional cell carcinoma of the bladder. European Urology. 2011;**60**(5):1066-1073

[38] Abreu AL, Chopra S, Dharmaraja A, Djaladat H, Aron M, Ukimura O, et al. Robot-assisted bladder diverticulectomy. Journal of Endourology. 2014;**28**(10): 1159-1164

[39] Schwentner C, Sim A, Balbay MD, Todenhofer T, Aufderklamm S, Halalsheh O, et al. Robot-assisted radical cystectomy and intracorporeal neobladder formation: On the way to a standardized procedure. World Journal of Surgical Oncology. 2015;**13**:3

[40] Sim A, Balbay MD, Todenhofer T, Aufderklamm S, Halalsheh O, Mischinger J, et al. Robot-assisted radical cystectomy and intracorporeal urinary diversion - safe and reproducible? Central European Journal of Urology. 2015;**68**(1):18-23

[41] Koie T, Ohyama C, Yoneyama T, Nagasaka H, Yamamoto H, Imai A, et al. Robotic cross-folded U-configuration intracorporeal ileal neobladder for muscle-invasive bladder cancer: Initial experience and functional outcomes. International Journal of Medical Robotics. 2018;**14**(6):e1955

[42] Desai MM, Gill IS, de Castro Abreu AL, Hosseini A, Nyberg T, Adding C, et al. Robotic intracorporeal orthotopic neobladder during radical cystectomy in 132 patients. The Journal of Urology. 2014;**192**(6):1734-1740

[43] Hussein AA, Ahmed YE, Kozlowski JD, May PR, Nyquist J, Sexton S, et al. Robot-assisted approach to 'W'-configuration urinary diversion: a step-by-step technique. BJU International. 2017;**120**(1):152-157

[44] Asimakopoulos AD, Campagna A, Gakis G, Corona Montes VE, Piechaud T, Hoepffner JL, et al. Nerve sparing, robot-assisted radical cystectomy with intracorporeal bladder substitution in the male. The Journal of Urology. 2016;**196**(5):1549-1557

[45] Checcucci E, Manfredi M, Sica M, Amparore D, De Cillis S, Volpi G, et al. Robot-assisted-radical-cystectomy with total intracorporeal Y neobladder: analysis of postoperative complications and functional outcomes with urodynamics findings. European Journal of Surgical Oncology. 2022;**48**(3):694-702

[46] Tan WS, Sridhar A, Goldstraw M, Zacharakis E, Nathan S, Hines J, et al. Robot-assisted intracorporeal pyramid neobladder. BJU International. 2015;**116**(5):771-779

[47] Simone G, Papalia R, Misuraca L, Tuderti G, Minisola F, Ferriero M, et al. Robotic intracorporeal padua ileal bladder: Surgical technique, perioperative, oncologic and functional outcomes. European Urology. 2018;**73**(6):934-940

[48] Cacciamani GE, De Marco V, Sebben M, Rizzetto R, Cerruto MA,

Porcaro AB, et al. Robot-assisted vescica ileale padovana: A new technique for intracorporeal bladder replacement reproducing open surgical principles. European Urology. 2019;**76**(3):381-390

[49] Minervini A, Vanacore D, Vittori G, Milanesi M, Tuccio A, Siena G, et al. Florence robotic intracorporeal neobladder (FloRIN): A new reconfiguration strategy developed following the IDEAL guidelines. BJU International. 2018;**121**(2):313-317

[50] Tyritzis SI, Hosseini A, Collins J, Nyberg T, Jonsson MN, Laurin O, et al. Oncologic, functional, and complications outcomes of robot-assisted radical cystectomy with totally intracorporeal neobladder diversion. European Urology. 2013;**64**(5):734-741

[51] Gok B, Atmaca AF, Canda AE, Asil E, Koc E, Ardicoglu A, et al. Robotic radical cystectomy with intracorporeal studer pouch formation for bladder cancer: experience in ninety-eight cases. Journal of Endourology. 2019;**33**(5):375-382

[52] Obrecht F, Youssef NA, Burkhardt O, Schregel C, Randazzo M, Padevit C, et al. Robot-assisted radical cystectomy and intracorporeal orthotopic neobladder: 1-year functional outcomes. Asian Journal of Andrology. 2020;**22**(2):145-148

[53] Mistretta FA, Musi G, Colla Ruvolo C, Conti A, Luzzago S, Catellani M, et al. Robot-assisted radical cystectomy for nonmetastatic urothelial carcinoma of urinary bladder: A comparison between intracorporeal versus extracorporeal orthotopic ileal neobladder. Journal of Endourology. 2021;**35**(2):151-158

Chapter 4

Review on Bladder Cancer Diagnosis

Sivapatham Sundaresan and S.K. Lavanya

Abstract

Urothelial bladder carcinoma (UBC) is the foremost as often as possible analyzed cancer of the bladder in men around the world, and it positioned the 6th in terms of the number of cases analyzed. A total 30% of bladder tumors likely result from word-related introduction within the work environment to carcinogens. Approximately 70–75% of recently analyzed UBCs are low-grade or non-invasive. As of 2019, there is insufficient evidence to determine whether or not screening bladder cancer in patients without symptoms is feasible. The determination of UBC is made utilizing distinctive tests such as pee cytology and cystoscopy. Cytology tests are uncaring for low-grade cancer, whereas cystoscopy measures the measure of the sore. A biopsy will be done in the event that anomalous tissue is found amid cystoscopy. UBC can be recognized early by cytology, which has moo affectability for low-grade cancer, and by cystoscopy, which is intrusive and costly. Subsequently, numerous analysts have meticulously distinguished pee natural markers for non-invasive UC determination so that treatment victory can be expanded. Organic markers for early UBC discovery are summarized in this chapter, counting FDA-approved and exploratory markers, as well as a few of the unused innovations and developments that have the potential to help investigate endeavors in early UC detection.

Keywords: biomarkers, cytology, diagnosis, urothelial bladder carcinoma, urine tumor markers, clinical utility

1. Introduction

Urothelial bladder cancer (UBC) has a high incidence and prevalence due to its indolent nature, with 1, 15, 949 and 17, 20, 625 cases in 2020 according to the WHO [1]. Among men, the incidence of UBC is three times greater than among women (3:1), making it the fourth most frequent malignancy among men. The main risk factors are age, smoking, chlorination by-products in drinking water, and occupational exposures [2].

Urothelial cancer recurrence and progression have yielded a molecular route that scientists are now investigating for predictive and prognostic indicators [3]. In addition, the emergence of new noninvasive detection and surveillance techniques as well as possible treatment targets has been facilitated [4]. While multi-institutional randomized prospective studies are lacking, however, their prognostic and predictive indicators have not yet been validated for regular clinical usage. A total of 80% of these studies are in the process of being developed or are being worked on and will revolutionize how we diagnose, assess, and treat cancers [5].

Non-muscle invasive urothelial tumors are believed to arise by at least two molecular routes, either high-grade papillary tumors or CIS. Low-grade and high-grade tumors have different mutations, but invasion tumors have different mutations. Because cancers are more likely to arise from premalignant urothelial cells, it is surprising that multifocal and metachronal tumors have both common and novel mutations [6]. Poorly differentiated invasive urothelial carcinoma tumors have been shown to be related to the growing degree of genomic instability and are prone to have low copy number variations and reductions in heterozygosity. Many tumor suppressor genes and oncogenes are thought to be involved in the development of invasive urothelial carcinoma (IUC), though it is frequently difficult to determine whether these factors are required. As a result, it is not surprising that multifocal and metachronal tumors have both common and novel mutations. [7].

This review discusses an update on bladder cancer diagnosis, including the currently available role of bladder cancer tumor producers, part of urine markers in early identification of bladder cancer, the role of tissue markers for prognosis, and part of urine markers for patient investigation.

2. Bladder cancer tumor makers

In the absence of disease-specific signs, the urologic community has struggled to diagnose and monitor bladder cancer patients. As the standard for bladder cancer detection, cystoscopy is invasive and costly, which limits its usage. Fluorescence and narrow-band imaging are two new technologies, but they come with invasiveness and extra costs that outweigh the need for them as diagnostic tools in light of better, easier, and less expensive tests for treating bladder cancer patients [8].

It is also important to consider the cost of these tests, especially when similar information may be obtained using less expensive routine exams (cytology, cystoscopy) or additional permitted biomarkers. Costs, the difficulty of performance, the interpretation made confusion in a specific clinical setting, and the “psychological stress” experienced by both patient and physician when evaluating the reliability of a test outcome should all be considered when applying any marker for “routine” clinical use due to the critical nature of establishing some “added value” in the use of a particular test.

However, the research design, period of follow-up, and numbers required to give statistical power in the direction to confirm results may be limited in such early publications. These factors, together with the misapplication of findings to diverse clinical settings, might explain the typical inability to confirm promising but preliminary results [9].

Urine screening of people who had smoked for 40 years or more, using a combination of UroVysion, cytology, and urinary dipstick testing for hematuria, revealed cancer in 3.3% of these high-risk people [10]. Similarly, combining microsatellite analysis of exfoliated urine with UroVysion FISH (Fluorescence *in situ* hybridization) and conventional urine cytology allowed for the identification of approximately 93% of patients with recurrent bladder cancer [11]. The presence of microsatellite changes in urine has a strong link to invasive tumors in the bladder and has a high sensitivity for individuals with invasive cancer.

A surprise biomarker for bladder cancer is urinary hematuria, which develops in 85% of patients. The effectiveness of urine dipstick tests conducted at home and followed by medical evaluation might range from 90 to 95%. Muscle invasion was seen in only 10% of newly diagnosed bladder cancer patients who were tested for hematuria at home, compared to 60% of newly diagnosed bladder cancer patients who were not tested for hematuria [12]. Overall mortality was also lower than in unscreened individuals. Unfortunately, hematuria only has a 0.08% positive predictive value [13]. The stratification of hematuria-positive individuals into low and high-risk categories is therefore urgently required.

Patients with bladder cancer who are diagnosed with non-muscle invasive illness will need to be monitored for the rest of their lives. Current patient-monitoring methods typically include cystoscopic examinations every 3 months for the first 2 years of follow-up, twice a year for years three and four, and then yearly until disease recurrence is detected.

3. Role of urine markers in early detection of bladder cancer

The Food and Drug Administration (FDA) has authorized the custom of many commercially available urine-based diagnostics. However, none of these tests are commonly performed and are not included in the clinical guidelines for BC therapy published by the American Urological Association or the European Association of Urology [14].

These multi-urinary protein indicators were found to be beneficial in both high- and low-grade illnesses, as well as high- and low-stage diseases [15]. Midkine (MDK) and synuclein G or MDK, ZAG2 and CEACAM1 [16], angiogenin and clusterin [17] are measured by immunoassay and urine cytology improves the sensitivity and specificity in the diagnosis of non-muscle invasive bladder cancer (NMIBC) [16].

In the urine sediments of NMIBC patients, higher amounts of CK20 and Insulin-Like Growth Factor II (IGFII) were originate compared to controls [18]. Improved urine HAI-1 and Epcam levels, as measured by ELISA, are predictive indicators in individuals with high-risk NMIBC [19]. Urinary survivin, as measured by a chemiluminescence enzyme immunoassay, is associated with tumor stage, lymph node, and distant metastases, and may be used as a preliminary marker for BC diagnosis [20]. In NMIBC, snail overexpression is a distinct prognostic marker for tumor recurrence [21]. Glycan-affinity glycoproteomics nano-platforms identified specific glycoproteins in the urine of low- and high-grade NMIBC patients; high-grade MIBC patients had greater urinary CD44 levels [22].

Metabolic profiling of urine may potentially be beneficial for early detection of bladder cancer. The very sensitive super-performance liquid chromatography and mass spectrometry confirmed the presence of imidazole-acetic acid in BC [23]. A metabolite panel that may distinguish high- and low-grade breast cancer by using indolylacryloyl glycine, N2-galacturonyl-L-lysine, and aspartyl-glutamate is possible [24]. Furthermore, UPLC-MS was used to show that the phenylalanine, arginine, proline, and tryptophan metabolisms had been altered in NMBIC.

Immunoassay and FISH testing have expanded the diagnostic armamentarium to help us decide who needs further investigation. The "liquid biopsy" test has recently been employed to distinguish between NMIBC and MIBC in urine by detecting exosomes, cell-free proteins/peptides, circulating cell-free DNA, DNA methylation, and miRNA, [25]. Advanced "nano-sensors" able to detect RNA and proteins in urine are becoming closer to reality. It is not far off from being something we could easily implement [26]. A practical solution is needed for those findings, however, studies to confirm the efficacy of the recently identified urine biomarkers are not available [27, 28].

4. Role of tissue markers for prognosis

Currently, the biggest challenge is translating substantial proteomic and genomic data into clinical practice and validating the expression of these biomarkers in well-designed multicenter clinical trials.

The biggest class of membrane proteins for signal transduction on the cell surface, G-protein-coupled receptors (GPCRs), is used to detect ligands of unknown identity [29]. More than 800 GPCRs are found in the human genome, with most of them including seven homologous transmembrane domains [30, 31]. To stimulate the movement of particular ligands, GPCRs alter their conformations by interacting with the ligands. After this, the signaling network will activate, producing cellular responses including erythroid differentiation [32]. The following is an excerpt from a 2013 study that reports that there are over 100 orphan G-protein-coupled receptors (oGPCRs) for which their respective ligands are yet unknown [33]. A gene that encodes a G protein-coupled receptor, GPR137, is expressed mostly in the central nervous system, endocrine glands, thymus, and lungs [34]. Studies have revealed that GPCRs are vital to tumor development and metastasis.

Various activities performed by GPCRs, such as cell proliferation, survival, and motility, have been documented [35]. The GPCR48 receptor was found to be associated with the growth of prostate cancer cells, making it a viable target for treating the disease [36]. Smith and colleagues discovered that GPR30 was expressed preferentially in high-risk epithelial ovarian cancer, a finding that has been shown to correlate with worse survival rates in patients [37]. In addition, GPR161 expression was found in breast cancer and an earlier investigation revealed that the gene is a major regulator and a possible therapeutic target for three-fold negative breast cancer [38].

In the area of bladder tumor marker testing, urine proteins are assessed qualitatively or quantitatively, and antigens or chromosomal abnormalities are detected in urine cytology samples. These tumor marker assays had better sensitivity for detecting urothelial carcinoma when compared to urine cytology. The overall sample's mean sensitivity and specificity were 64–80% and 71–95%, respectively, while the mean positive predictive value (PPV) and negative predictive value (NPV) for malignancy classification were 49–84% and 79–95%, respectively. During studies identifying proteins secreted into urine by bladder cancer cells, sensitivity was inadequate for Ta grade 1 bladder cancer. Since there are so many false-positive results with BTA TRAK, BTA stat, NMP22, and NMP22 Bladder Chek assays in patients with benign urological diseases like hematuria, urocystitis, renal calculi, or UTIs, as well as in patients with inserted catheters or intravesical manipulation in the last weeks, these tests are unreliable in these populations. If you are investigating a problem with BTA TRAK, BTA stat, NMP22, or NMP22 BladderChek, you must first eliminate other possible diagnoses, such as benign or malignant genitourinary illness, except for bladder cancer. The failure of urine tests to accurately diagnose bladder cancer or to be relied upon to guide treatment choice leads to a lack of appropriate sensitivity and specificity [39].

CD164, a member of the sialomucin family and previously known as endolyn or MGC-24v, was located on human chromosome 6q21 and is expressed and encoded by the CD164 gene [40, 41]. CD164 was originally discovered in primitive CD34+ hemopoietic progenitor cells and bone marrow stromal cells and is now known to have a role in adhesion, migration, and cell proliferation [42–44]. CD164, which was hypothesized to control hematopoiesis, was thought to have a role in promoting the adherence and migration of human CD34+ cells to bone marrow stroma [45].

A variety of malignancies in humans are known to have CD164 perform various functions. CD164, for example, has been documented for maintaining and progressing human malignancies, such as human glioma [46], lung cancer [47], ovarian cancer [48], and prostate cancer [49].

5. Role of urine markers for patient surveillance

Improved sequencing technology and a greater understanding of the molecular mechanisms of action for various treatments have both aided the study of BC tumor biology and how it affects MIBC and NMIBC. However, there are no clinically useful biomarkers available to accurately predict response to therapy in either the short- or long-term. An in-depth understanding of the clinicopathological parameters, such as tumor stage, grade, presence of CIS, tumor size, tumor multiplicity, and recurrence, is essential to properly predict treatment outcomes [50]. It was demonstrated that recurrence could be predicted with 85.5% accuracy using a cytokine panel after intravesical therapy (CyPRIT) (IL-2, IL-8, IL-6, IL-Ira, IL-18, IL-12), Il-12, tumour necrosis factor-, and tumour necrosis factor-, but its validity needed to be confirmed.

New discoveries related to the immunologic characteristics of bladder cancer (BC) have emerged as a promising prediction tool for intravesical BCG treatment and possibly immunotherapy in advanced cases [51]. While some studies found no link between programmed cell death protein ligand 1 (PDL-1) expression and the outcomes of NMIBC following BCG administration, others reported contradictory results and no convincing evidence [52]. It has been shown that an improved clinical result can be achieved by the assessment of BCG-specific T-cell immunity [53, 54]. In a study of BCG therapy, the T-cell and MDSC ratio in urine was associated with treatment failure [55].

A number of writers have attempted to find genetic alterations that might be associated with a response to the BCG vaccine. One example is the ARID1A mutation, which was found to increase the likelihood of BCG unresponsiveness [56]. Even while we now have non-invasive diagnostic tests and sensitive and specialized follow-up tests, our systems are still plagued by troublesome false positive findings. In addition to the presence of benign diseases including hematuria, cystitis, lithiasis, urinary tract infections, inflammation, and recurrent instrumentation, such as cystoscopy, false positive rates can develop due to many other reasons. Regardless, many kits have been on the market for quite some time. Even if most non-invasive techniques are better than standard cytology, this is not a hazard because of this superior performance. Due to the fact that none of these kits meet all requirements at all phases of BC detection, they have not yet been adopted in clinical practice. Patients and healthcare providers can benefit from each kit based on patient characteristics, context, and limits in detecting BC. Patients stratification is a crucial biological topic that is being addressed by the development of new biomarkers that can predict disease recurrence and response to medication. To be sure, cell-free (cfDNA) analysis in urine and/or serum will be able to overcome these barriers when liquid biopsies and precision oncology become more common [57].

Even for higher-grade bladder cancer, a number of molecular markers surpass urine cytology with regard to test sensitivity, as suggested by marker performance assessment. The cause of the decline in performance quality among pathologists is not known, however, it might be that it is caused by a reduction in urine cytology during the previous decade. The decreased specificity of molecular markers in the group studied seems insignificant because the priority is sensitivity when tracking individuals with high-grade malignancies. A further query is if at least some of the false-positive results may be an anticipatory positive finding, forecasting tumor recurrence [58, 59]. Studies indicating that molecular markers may improve the prognosis of bladder cancer patients with high-grade tumors are lacking, thus they are not widely accepted for therapeutic usage.

The vast array of mutations found in bladder cancer cases was revealed by a series of studies on next-generation sequencing, which found that more than 300 mutations were identified in each tumor, with 200 copy number changes and 20 rearrangements. Despite having a higher mutation rate, the only kind of cancer that has been found to have more mutations is lung cancer, and most of them are considered to be passenger mutations that have no effect [60].

A discussion on the clinical risk of recurrence and progression is, of course, ongoing, and several factors are in play, but largely because recurrence and advancement are both dictated by the presence of characteristics including size, multimodality, and time to recurrence. In addition, we must recognize that grading is primarily subjective and will, in the future, lead to increased reproducibility and improved association with a clinical result (either immunohistochemistry or molecular testing [61]. Hyperplasia was made obsolete when the phrase urothelial proliferation with undetermined malignant potential was established [62, 63]. The urothelium is thicker with few or no cytological abnormalities and a lack of genuine papillary fronds, however, undulations are sometimes present. These features may be observed in this context without any known history. When previous cancer or papillary lesions are present, those with carcinoma tend to have them. Lateral expansion of papillary carcinoma is expected, with high rates of chromosome 9 deletions and lower but still substantial rates of FGFR3 abnormalities. A flat lesion with cytologic and architectural abnormalities that are thought to be preneoplastic but do not meet the requirements for urothelial CIS is known as urothelial dysplasia. Because it seldom arises de novo, it is not well investigated. Of greater significance, this is the most difficult group to characterize morphologically because of a substantial inter-observer variability and a total lack of major clinical trials demonstrating its association with the later development of CIS.

6. Conclusion

The wide range of bladder cancer indicators enhances the prospect of making a breakthrough in the detection of cancer by using chosen markers, either in combination or individually. Hence panel testing is useful for increasing the detection of bladder cancer as well as for enhancing the accuracy of that detection. It is unquestionably crucial to test the clinical usefulness of this kind of panel before it can be used in standard medical treatment. The stability of these tumor marker analytes should also be better characterized in order to avoid false negative findings. A greater understanding of circumstances that result in false positives for urine-based indicators for cancer diagnosis might make them more effective.

Author details

Sivapatham Sundaresan* and S.K. Lavanya
Department of Medical Research, SRM Medical College Hospital and Research Centre, SRM Institute of Science and Technology, SRM Nagar, Kattankalathur, Tamil Nadu, India

*Address all correspondence to: ssunsrm@gmail.com

References

[1] Ferlay J, Shin HR, Bray F, Forman D, Mathers C, Parkin DM. Estimates of worldwide burden of cancer in 2008: GLOBOCAN 2008. International Journal of Cancer. 2010;**127**(12):2893-2917

[2] Murta-Nascimento C, Schmitz-Dräger BJ, Zeegers MP, Steineck G, Kogevinas M, Real FX, et al. Epidemiology of urinary bladder cancer: From tumor development to patient's death. World Journal of Urology. 2007;**25**(3):285-295

[3] Nordentoft I, Lamy P, Birkenkamp-Demtröder K, Shumansky K, Vang S, Hornshøj H, et al. Mutational context and diverse clonal development in early and late bladder cancer. Cell Reports. 2014;7(5):1649-1663

[4] Netto GJ. Molecular biomarkers in urothelial carcinoma of the bladder: Are we there yet? Nature Reviews Urology. 2012;**9**(1):41

[5] Readal N, Epstein JI. Papillary urothelial hyperplasia: Relationship to urothelial neoplasms. Pathology. 2010;**42**(4):360-363

[6] Nordentoft I, Lamy P, Birkenkamp-Demtröder K, Shumansky K, Vang S, Hornshøj H, et al. Mutational context and diverse clonal development in early and late bladder cancer. Cell Reports. 2014;7(5):1649-1663

[7] Knowles MA. Molecular subtypes of bladder cancer: Jekyll and Hyde or chalk and cheese? Carcinogenesis. 2006;**27**(3):361-373

[8] Shariat SF, Lotan Y, Vickers A, Karakiewicz PI, Schmitz-Dräger BJ, Goebell PJ, Malats N. Statistical consideration for clinical biomarker research in bladder cancer. In Urologic Oncology: Seminars and Original Investigations 2010 28, 4, pp. 389-400. Elsevier.

[9] Schmitz-Dräger BJ, Droller M, Lokeshwar VB, Lotan Y, M'Liss AH, Van Rhijn BW, et al. Molecular markers for bladder cancer screening, early diagnosis, and surveillance: The WHO/ICUD consensus. Urologia Internationalis. 2015;**94**(1):1-24

[10] Steiner H, Bergmeister M, Verdorfer I, Granig T, Mikuz G, Bartsch G, et al. Early results of bladder-cancer screening in a high-risk population of heavy smokers. BJU International. 2008;**102**(3):291-296

[11] Frigerio S, Padberg BC, Strebel RT, Lenggenhager DM, Messthaler A, Abdou MT, et al. Improved detection of bladder carcinoma cells in voided urine by standardized microsatellite analysis. International Journal of Cancer. 2007;**121**(2):329-338

[12] Messing EM, Madeb R, Young T, Gilchrist KW, Bram L, Greenberg EB, et al. Long-term outcome of hematuria home screening for bladder cancer in men. Cancer: Interdisciplinary International Journal of the American Cancer Society. 2006;**107**(9):2173-2179

[13] Messing EM, Young TB, Hunt VB, Gilchrist KW, Newton MA, Bram LL, et al. Comparison of bladder cancer outcome in men undergoing hematuria home screening versus those with standard clinical presentations. Urology. 1995;**45**(3):387-397

[14] Zuiverloon TC, de Jong FC, Theodorescu D. Clinical decision making in surveillance of non–muscle-invasive

bladder cancer: The evolving roles of urinary cytology and molecular markers. Oncology. 2017;**31**(12):855-862

[15] Masuda N, Ogawa O, Park M, Liu AY, Goodison S, Dai Y, et al. Meta-analysis of a 10-plex urine-based biomarker assay for the detection of bladder cancer. Oncotarget. 2018;**9**(6):7101

[16] Soukup V, Kalousová M, Capoun O, Sobotka R, Breyl Z, Pešl M, et al. Panel of urinary diagnostic markers for non-invasive detection of primary and recurrent urothelial urinary bladder carcinoma. Urologia Internationalis. 2015;**95**(1):56-64

[17] Shabayek MI, Sayed OM, Attaia HA, Awida HA, Abozeed H. Diagnostic evaluation of urinary angiogenin (ANG) and clusterin (CLU) as biomarker for bladder cancer. Pathology & Oncology Research. 2014;**20**(4):859-866

[18] Salomo K, Huebner D, Boehme MU, Herr A, Brabetz W, Heberling U, et al. Urinary transcript quantitation of CK20 and IGF2 for the non-invasive bladder cancer detection. Journal of Cancer Research and Clinical Oncology. 2017;**143**(9):1757-1769

[19] Snell KI, Ward DG, Gordon NS, Goldsmith JC, Sutton AJ, Patel P, et al. Exploring the roles of urinary HAI-1, EpCAM & EGFR in bladder cancer prognosis & risk stratification. Oncotarget. 2018;**9**(38):25244

[20] Yang Y, Xu J, Zhang Q. Detection of urinary survivin using a magnetic particles-based chemiluminescence immunoassay for the preliminary diagnosis of bladder cancer and renal cell carcinoma combined with LAPTM4B. Oncology Letters. 2018;**15**(5):7923-7933

[21] Santi R, Cai T, Nobili S, Galli IC, Amorosi A, Comperat E, et al. Snail immunohistochemical overexpression correlates to recurrence risk in non-muscle invasive bladder cancer: Results from a longitudinal cohort study. Virchows Archiv. 2018;**472**(4):605-613

[22] Azevedo R, Soares J, Gaiteiro C, Peixoto A, Lima L, Ferreira D, et al. Glycan affinity magnetic nanoplatforms for urinary glycobiomarkers discovery in bladder cancer. Talanta. 2018;**184**:347-355

[23] Shao CH, Chen CL, Lin JY, Chen CJ, Fu SH, Chen YT, et al. Metabolite marker discovery for the detection of bladder cancer by comparative metabolomics. Oncotarget. 2017;**8**(24):38802

[24] Liu X, Cheng X, Liu X, He L, Zhang W, Wang Y, et al. Investigation of the urinary metabolic variations and the application in bladder cancer biomarker discovery. International Journal of Cancer. 2018;**143**(2):408-418

[25] Ward DG, Bryan RT. Liquid biopsies for bladder cancer. Translational Andrology and Urology. 2017;**6**(2):331

[26] Wald C. Diagnostics: A flow of information. Nature. 2017;**551**:S48-S50

[27] Piao XM, Byun YJ, Kim WJ, Kim J. Unmasking molecular profiles of bladder cancer. Investigative and Clinical Urology. 2018;**59**(2):72-82

[28] Soria F, Droller MJ, Lotan Y, Gontero P, D'Andrea D, Gust KM, et al. An up-to-date catalog of available urinary biomarkers for the surveillance of non-muscle invasive bladder cancer. World Journal of Urology. 2018;**36**(12):1981-1995

[29] Vanti WB, Nguyen T, Cheng R, Lynch KR, George SR, O'Dowd BF. Novel human G-protein-coupled receptors. Biochemical and Biophysical Research Communications. 2003;**305**(1):67-71

[30] Łazarczyk M, Matyja E, Lipkowski A. Substance P and its receptors–a potential target for novel medicines in malignant brain tumor therapies (mini-review). Folia Neuropathologica. 2007;**45**(3):99-107

[31] Pierce KL, Premont RT, Lefkowitz RJ. Seven-transmembrane receptors. Nature Reviews Molecular Cell Biology. 2002;**3**(9):639-650

[32] Rosenbaum DM, Rasmussen SG, Kobilka BK. The structure and function of G-protein-coupled receptors. Nature. 2009;**459**(7245):356-363

[33] Yoshida M, Miyazato M, Kangawa K. Orphan GPCRs and methods for identifying their ligands. In Methods in Enzymology 2012 Vol. 514, pp. 33-44. Academic Press.

[34] Regard JB, Sato IT, Coughlin SR. Anatomical profiling of G protein-coupled receptor expression. Cell. 2008;**135**(3):561-571

[35] Dorsam RT, Gutkind JS. G-protein-coupled receptors and cancer. Nature Reviews Cancer. 2007;**7**(2):79-94

[36] Liang F, Yue J, Wang J, Zhang L, Fan R, Zhang H, et al. GPCR48/LGR4 promotes tumorigenesis of prostate cancer via PI3K/Akt signaling pathway. Medical Oncology. 2015;**32**(3):49

[37] Smith HO, Arias-Pulido H, Kuo DY, Howard T, Qualls CR, Lee SJ, et al. GPR30 predicts poor survival for ovarian cancer. Gynecologic Oncology. 2009;**114**(3):465-471

[38] Feigin ME, Xue B, Hammell MC, Muthuswamy SK. G-protein–coupled receptor GPR161 is overexpressed in breast cancer and is a promoter of cell proliferation and invasion. Proceedings of the National Academy of Sciences. 2014;**111**(11):4191-4196

[39] Stenzl A, Feil G. Tumor markers in bladder cancer. European Oncology Review. 2005:1-7

[40] Watt SM, Bühring HJ, Rappold I, Chan JY, Lee-Prudhoe J, Jones T, et al. CD164, a novel sialomucin on CD34+ and erythroid subsets, is located on human chromosome 6q21. Blood, The Journal of the American Society of Hematology. 1998;**92**(3):849-866

[41] Kurosawa N, Kanemitsu Y, Matsui T, Shimada K, Ishihama H, Muramatsu T. Genomic analysis of a murine cell-surface sialomucin, MGC-24/CD164. European Journal of Biochemistry. 1999;**265**(1):466-472

[42] Watt SM, Butler LH, Tavian M, Bühring HJ, Rappold I, Simmons PJ, et al. Functionally defined CD164 epitopes are expressed on CD34+ cells throughout ontogeny but display distinct distribution patterns in adult hematopoietic and nonhematopoietic tissues. Blood, The Journal of the American Society of Hematology. 2000;**95**(10):3113-3124

[43] Doyonnas R, Chan JY, Butler LH, RappoldI,Lee-PrudhoeJE,ZannettinoAC, et al. CD164 monoclonal antibodies that block hemopoietic progenitor cell adhesion and proliferation interact with the first mucin domain of the CD164 receptor. The Journal of Immunology. 2000;**165**(2):840-851

[44] Zannettino AC, Bühring HJ, Niutta S, Watt SM, Benton MA, Simmons PJ. The sialomucin CD164 (MGC-24v) is an adhesive glycoprotein expressed by human hematopoietic progenitors and bone marrow stromal cells that serves as a potent negative regulator of hematopoiesis. Blood, The Journal of the American Society of Hematology. 1998;**92**(8):2613-2628

[45] Ihrke G, Gray SR, Luzio JP. Endolyn is a mucin-like type I membrane

protein targeted to lysosomes by its cytoplasmic tail. Biochemical Journal. 2000;**345**(2):287-296

[46] Tu M, Cai L, Zheng W, Su Z, Chen Y, Qi S. CD164 regulates proliferation and apoptosis by targeting PTEN in human glioma. Molecular Medicine Reports. 2017;**15**(4):1713-1721

[47] Chen WL, Huang AF, Huang SM, Ho CL, Chang YL, Chan JY. CD164 promotes lung tumor-initiating cells with stem cell activity and determines tumor growth and drug resistance via Akt/mTOR signaling. Oncotarget. 2017;**8**(33):54115

[48] Huang AF, Chen MW, Huang SM, Kao CL, Lai HC, Chan JY. CD164 regulates the tumorigenesis of ovarian surface epithelial cells through the SDF-1α/CXCR4 axis. Molecular Cancer. 2013;**12**(1):1-3

[49] Havens AM, Jung Y, Sun YX, Wang J, Shah RB, Bühring HJ, et al. The role of sialomucin CD164 (MGC-24v or endolyn) in prostate cancer metastasis. BMC Cancer. 2006;**6**(1):195

[50] Xylinas E, Kent M, Kluth L, Pycha A, Comploj E, Svatek RS, et al. Accuracy of the EORTC risk tables and of the CUETO scoring model to predict outcomes in non-muscle-invasive urothelial carcinoma of the bladder. British Journal of Cancer. 2013;**109**(6):1460-1466

[51] Kamat AM, Briggman J, Urbauer DL, Svatek R, González GM, Anderson R, et al. Cytokine panel for response to intravesical therapy (CyPRIT): Nomogram of changes in urinary cytokine levels predicts patient response to bacillus Calmette-Guérin. European Urology. 2016;**69**(2):197-200

[52] Wankowicz SA, Werner L, Orsola A, Novak J, Bowden M, Choueiri TK, et al. Differential expression of PD-L1 in high grade T1 vs muscle invasive bladder carcinoma and its prognostic implications. The Journal of Urology. 2017;**198**(4):817-823

[53] Luftenegger W, Ackermann DK, Futterlieb A, Kraft R, Minder CE, Nadelhaft P, et al. Intravesical versus intravesical plus intradermal bacillus Calmette-Guerin: A prospective randomized study in patient with recurrent superficial bladder tumors. The Journal of Urology. 1996;**155**(2):483-487

[54] Saint F, Salomon L, Quintela R, Cicco A, Hoznek A, Abbou CC, et al. Do prognostic parameters of remission versus relapse after bacillus Calmette–Guérin (BCG) immunotherapy exist?: Analysis of a quarter century of literature. European Urology. 2003;**43**(4):351-361

[55] Chevalier MF, Trabanelli S, Racle J, Salomé B, Cesson V, Gharbi D, et al. ILC2-modulated T cell–to-MDSC balance is associated with bladder cancer recurrence. The Journal of Clinical Investigation. 2017;**127**(8):2916-2929

[56] Pietzak EJ, Bagrodia A, Cha EK, Drill EN, Iyer G, Isharwal S, et al. Next-generation sequencing of nonmuscle invasive bladder cancer reveals potential biomarkers and rational therapeutic targets. European Urology. 2017;**72**(6):952-959

[57] Batista R, Vinagre N, Meireles S, Vinagre J, Prazeres H, Leão R, et al. Biomarkers for bladder cancer diagnosis and surveillance: A comprehensive review. Diagnostics. 2020;**10**(1):39

[58] Yoder BJ, Skacel M, Hedgepeth R, Babineau D, Ulchaker JC, Liou LS, et al. Reflex UroVysion testing of bladder cancer surveillance patients with equivocal or negative urine cytology:

A prospective study with focus on the natural history of anticipatory positive findings. American Journal of Clinical Pathology. 2007;**127**(2):295-301

[59] Skacel M, Fahmy M, Brainard JA, Pettay JD, Biscotti CV, Liou LS, et al. Multitarget fluorescence in situ hybridization assay detects transitional cell carcinoma in the majority of patients with bladder cancer and atypical or negative urine cytology. The Journal of Urology. 2003;**169**(6):2101-2105

[60] Balbás-Martínez C, Sagrera A, Carrillo-de-Santa-Pau E, Earl J, Márquez M, Vazquez M, et al. Recurrent inactivation of STAG2 in bladder cancer is not associated with aneuploidy. Nature Genetics. 2013;**45**(12):1464-1469

[61] Guo G, Sun X, Chen C, Wu S, Huang P, Li Z, et al. Whole-genome and whole-exome sequencing of bladder cancer identifies frequent alterations in genes involved in sister chromatid cohesion and segregation. Nature Genetics. 2013;**45**(12):1459-1463

[62] Kandoth C, McLellan MD, Vandin F, Ye K, Niu B, Lu C, et al. Mutational landscape and significance across 12 major cancer types. Nature. 2013;**502**(7471):333-339

[63] Kim PH, Cha EK, Sfakianos JP, Iyer G, Zabor EC, Scott SN, et al. Genomic predictors of survival in patients with high-grade urothelial carcinoma of the bladder. European Urology. 2015;**67**(2):198-201

Chapter 5

A Rare but Real Entity: Bladder Neuroendocrine Cancer

Béla Pikó, Ali Bassam, Anita Kis, Paul Ovidiu Rus-Gal, Ibolya Laczó and Tibor Mészáros

Abstract

The neuoroendocrine cancer of the bladder is a rare tumour, and from this entity the well-differentiated tumours with favourable prognosis, the paraganglioma with unfavourable prognosis, small and large cell types of tumours should be emphasised. From the methods of the anticancer therapies' operation can be eligible by itself in the first group but in the second group should form only the part of the multimodal treatment. Radiotherapy plays a role only in the treatment of the small and large cell tumours, and during the treatment of these tumours, the administration of the cytostatic drugs is also essential (mainly platina derivates). Somatostatin analogues, immune checkpoint inhibitors could be beneficial in special cases and some tumour agnostic treatment can be useful as well. Moreover, the palliative treatment should represent an important modality even in the early treatment period, but it should also be provided when no other treatment options are left.

Keywords: neuroendocrine tumour of the bladder, operation, radiotherapy and medical therapy, tumour agnostic therapy, palliative treatment

1. Introduction

Bladder cancer is not one of the most common tumours (**Table 1**) [1–3]. The prevalence of neuroendocrine bladder cancer (NEBC) in muscle invasive processes is estimated to be 0.5–1.2% [4], while others estimate it to be less than 1% [5, 6]. The statistically expected 5700 (in Hungarian only 35) patients with various common symptoms—haematuria, pelvic pain, urinary obstruction—are detected and diagnosed in urological centres and efficient onco-teams (multidisciplinary teams) give them the chance to receive adequate treatment [7–10]. However, these tumours require special attention because they usually have a poor prognosis, undifferentiated forms are usually detected at a disseminated stage, and their treatment differs from the usual treatment for bladder cancer [8, 11].

	incidence (new cases)		mortality	
	males	females	males	females
all cancers (excluding non-melanoma skin cancer) [1]	4,824,700	4,110,118	1,926,292	1,552,475
of these bladder cancer [2]	440,864	132,414	158,785	53,751
bladder cancer in Hungary [3]	2393	1132	706	392

Table 1.
Incidence and mortality all cancers and bladder cancer [1–3].

2. Pathology

The WHO pathological classification is shown in **Table 2** [12]. The tumours can be differentiated in different ways, the well-differentiated form is extremely rare and, according to the literature, is usually not associated with carcinoid symptoms and has one of the best prognoses. Small cell NEBC is the most common, although the 'pure' form is rare, with more than half of cases (up to 61% according to some authors) being associated with transitional cell bladder cancer, glandular or squamous cell carcinoma, possibly with a sarcomatoid component, and is more common in women. Large cell tumours are also rare and, like small cell tumours, have a poor prognosis. Paragangliomas can also occur in the bladder, usually described in case reports; interestingly, they can be functional (producing catecholamines), with the 'usual'

(Listing neuroendrocrine tumours in details)
Urothelial tumours
Infiltrating urothelial tumours
Non-invasive urothelial tumours
Squamous cell neoplasms
Glandular neoplasms
Urachal carcinoma
Tumours of Müllerian type
Neuroendocrine tumours
Small cell neuroendocrine carcinoma
Large cell neuroendocrine carcinoma
Well-differentiated neuroendocrine tumour
Paraganglioma
Melanocytic tumours
Mesenchymal tumours
Urothelial tract haematopoietic and lymphoid tumours
Miscellaneous tumours

Table 2.
WHO classification of tumours of the urothelial tract [12].

clinical symptoms (sudden spikes in blood pressure, possibly hypertension, headache, palpitations, sweating, visual disturbances) caused by bladder distension or contractions. Survival data are relatively favourable, as far as it can be concluded from only a few patients [6, 13–18].

3. Diagnosis

Based on the symptoms, the clinical and imaging methods used to diagnose NEBC are the ones commonly used for bladder cancer and reported in other publications in this volume. Accurate pathological diagnosis is essential, but it is not within our competence. In the light of the histological findings, the need for axial imaging techniques—CT and MR—to assess the small cell form progression is highlighted in the literature, and bone scintigraphy is necessary in the case of osteoarticular complaints but should also be considered in the absence of symptoms [8, 19, 20]. In functional paragangliomas, MIBG (iodine-123 meta-iodobenzylguanidine) scintigraphy and PET/CT can indicate local expansion and possible distant metastases with up to 95% accuracy [16].

4. Treatment and prognosis

As there are only a few cases and thus clinical trial results with high evidence level are not available, the therapeutic recommendations are based on a summary of institutional experience and partly on analogies to the treatment of other neuroendocrine tumours. Early detection of the disease, its progression, accurate diagnosis and good overall patient health (ECOG PS [Eastern Cooperative Oncology Group Performance Status]) improve outcomes. In general, even with a carefully chosen and correctly executed treatment, the prognosis depends mainly on the differentiation of the tumour: favourable in well-differentiated NEBC and paraganglioma, unfavourable in small and large cell tumours [6, 11, 13, 15–17].

4.1 Surgery

A biopsy during cystoscopy is almost always necessary [8, 13]. For well-differentiated NEBC and paraganglioma, adequately radical surgery (partial or radical cystectomy) may be a solution in itself but for functionally active tumours, pre-operative endocrinological consultation and medication are essential. In small- and large-cell forms, surgery (depending on the dissemination status) may be considered as part of a complex treatment, and although significance is questionable due to the small number of cases in these studies, it seems that surgery in selected cases may improve survival [13, 15–17].

4.2 Radiotherapy

It can be an alternative to surgery in exceptional cases of well-differentiated forms and paragangliomas and applied to treat local recurrences. In paraganglioma, ^{131}I MIBG treatment has a beneficial effect on symptoms. For small and large cell NEBC, radiotherapy is an essential part of multimodality treatment. The recommendation of the Canadian Association of Genitourinary Medical Oncologists (CAGMO) includes prophylactic cranial irradiation and—as appropriate—irradiation of symptomatic metastases [5, 6, 8, 11, 13, 15, 21].

4.3 Somatostatin receptor analogues

In functional forms of differentiated NEBC—their use, as in other neuroendocrine tumours—is logical and results in symptom relief (due to the small number of cases, anti-tumour effects cannot be assessed) [22–24].

4.4 Cytostatic treatment

Its role is minor in well-differentiated tumours. In this regard, small- and large-cell NEBC can be grouped together in practice, since in these cases cytostatic treatment is considered both as neoadjuvant or adjuvant treatment and as part of radiochemotherapy, and in disseminated disease it is almost the only option. Whether used alone or as part of a multimodal regimen, from cytostatics cisplatin (or possibly carboplatin) and etoposide, ifosfamide-doxorubicin, cisplatin (or carboplatin) and irinotecan are recommended, and in mixed tumours, methotrexate, vincristine, cyclophosphamide and taxanes may be added. The poor general condition of the patient sometimes only allows monotherapy [5, 8, 11, 13, 16, 17, 21, 25–29].

4.5 Immune checkpoint inhibitors

PD-1 (programmed cell death protein 1) and PD-L1 (programmed death-ligand 1) inhibitors have also been tested in this disorder, and although they have generally not been successful, positive results have been described in case reports. Clinical trials with adequate evidence are ongoing [11, 30–32].

4.6 Tumour-agnostic treatment

The 'classical' knowledge of tumours includes the organ origin, histological structure, tumour infiltration, differentiation, prognostic and predictive markers, etc., while the agnostic approach does not consider these as essential but focuses on the genetic target of treatment. Drugs acting on targets in tumour-agnostic treatment have a convincing anti-tumour effect regardless of the organ of origin, meaning that detection of the target (often by genetic testing) is highly likely to predict treatment success. Currently, three drugs and three targets in NEBC can meet these requirements, as specified by the European and North American Medicines Agency. These: pembrolizumab (EMA [European Medicines Agency] and FDA [U. S. Food and Drug Administration] for PD-L1, MSI-H [Microsatellite Instability high] and dMMR [DNA mismatch repair deficiency]), larotrectinib, (both EMA and FDA for NTRK [Neurotrophic tyrosine receptor kinase] gene fusion) and entrectinib EMA and FDA for NTRK gene fusion or ROS-1 (Proto-oncogene tyrosine-protein kinase 1) positive non-small-cell lung cancer [33–42].

5. Palliative and terminal care

According to the WHO (World Health Organisation) definition, 'Palliative care is a crucial part of integrated, people-centred health services. Relieving serious health-related suffering, be it physical, psychological, social, or spiritual, is a global ethical responsibility. Thus, whether the cause of suffering is cardiovascular disease, cancer, major organ failure, drug-resistant tuberculosis, severe burns, end-stage chronic illness, acute trauma, extreme birth prematurity or extreme frailty of old age, palliative care may be needed and must be available at all levels of care' [43]. This includes curative anticancer treatment and symptomatic therapy (drugs, physiotherapy, psychosocial support, terminal care, ensuring a dignified death and dealing with the grief response if needed). In well-established oncology centres, some elements of early palliation have always been used and are still used, but the biggest problem is the period after active treatment options run out when due to limited capacity, a large proportion of patients are discharged from the care system. For NEBC, in addition to the necessary pain relief, management of functioning tumour symptoms, management of catheters and drains, athropia, anaemia, incontinence, bleeding from the bladder, painful, crampy urination, possible pelvic compression symptoms and body image changes and depression after advanced surgery are also problems to be addressed [44–47].

Acknowledgements

We would like to thank the editorial staff of the journal Hungarian Oncology ('Magyar Onkológia') for contributing to the processing of our publication—'A rare but real entity: bladder neuroendocrine cancer' (Magy Onkol. 65:355–358, 2021. [With English abstract])—entitled.

Conflict of interest

The authors declare no conflict of interest.

Author details

Béla Pikó*, Ali Bassam, Anita Kis, Paul Ovidiu Rus-Gal, Ibolya Laczó and Tibor Mészáros
Pándy Kálmán Hospital, Member of the Békés County Central Hospital, Centre of Oncology, Gyula, Hungary

*Address all correspondence to: dr.piko.bela@gmail.com

References

[1] World Health Organization International Agency for Research on Cancer. All cancers excluding non-melanoma skin cancer. Source: Globocan. 2020 [Internet] https://gco.iarc.fr/today/data/factsheets/cancers/40-All-cancers-excluding-non-melanoma-skin-cancer-fact-sheet.pdf. [Accessed: 2022-06-08]

[2] World Health Organization International Agency for Research on Cancer. Bladder. Source: Globocan. 2020 [Internet] https://gco.iarc.fr/today/data/factsheets/cancers/30-Bladder-fact-sheet.pdf. [Accessed: 2022-06-08]

[3] Bladder Cancer. Data. 2017. Source: KSH (Central Statistics Office, Reported cancer patients. In Hungarian language.) [Internet] https://www.ksh.hu/stadat_files/ege/hu/ege0025.html. [Accessed: 2022-06-08]

[4] Batista da Costa J, Gibb EA, Bivalacqua TJ, Liu Y, Oo HZ, Miyamoto DT, et al. Mint: Molecular characterization of neuroendocrine-like bladder cancer. Clinical Cancer Research. 2019;**25**(13):3908-3920. DOI: 10.1158/1078-0432.CCR-18-3558

[5] Xia K, Zhong W, Chen J, Lai Y, Huang G, et al. Mint: Clinical characteristics, treatment strategy, and outcomes of primary large cell neuroendocrine carcinoma of the bladder: A case report and systematic review of the literature. Frontiers in Oncology. 2020;**10**:1291. DOI: 10.3389/fonc.2020.01291

[6] Niu Q, Lu Y, Xu S, Shi Q, Guo B, et al. Mint: Clinicopathological characteristics and survival outcomes of bladder neuroendocrine carcinomas: A population-based study. Mint: Cancer Management and Research. 2018;**10**:4479-4489. DOI: 10.2147/CMAR.S175286

[7] Fotopoulos G, Pentheroudakis G, Ioachim E, Pavlidis N. Mint: A patient with neuroendocrine carcinoma of the urinary bladder and paraneoplastic degenerative parencephalitis: A case report and review of the literature. Cancer Treatment Communications. 2014;**2**(1):8-11. DOI: 10.1016/J.CTRC.2013.12.001

[8] Masood B, Iqbal N, Iqbal W, Masood Y, Akbar MK, et al. Mint: Small-cell neuroendocrine carcinoma of the urinary bladder: A case report. International Journal of Health Sciences (Qassim). 2020;**14**(2):53-55. PMID: 32206060; PMCID: PMC7069666.

[9] Lamb BW, Jalil RT, Sevdalis N, Vincent C, Green JS. Mint: Strategies to improve the efficiency and utility of multidisciplinary team meetings in urology cancer care: A survey study. BMC Health Services Research. 2014;**14**:377. DOI: 10.1186/1472-6963-14-377

[10] Askelin B, Hind A, Paterson C. Mint: Exploring the impact of uro-oncology multidisciplinary team meetings on patient outcomes: A systematic review. European Journal of Oncology Nursing. 2021;**54**:102032. DOI: 10.1016/j.ejon.2021.102032

[11] Flaig TW, Spiess PE, Abern M, Agarwal N, Bangs R, et al. Mint: NCCN Clinical Practice Guidelines in Oncology (NCCN Guidelines®). Bladder Cancer. Version 2.2022 — May 20, 2022 [Internet] https://www.nccn.org/professionals/physician_gls/pdf/bladder.pdf. [Accessed: 2022-06-01]

[12] Humphrey PA, Moch H, Cubilla AL, Ulbright TM, et al. Mint: The 2016 WHO

classification of tumours of the urinary system and male genital organs-Part B: Prostate and bladder tumours. European Urology. 2016;**70**(1):106-119. DOI: 10.1016/j.eururo.2016.02.028

[13] Pósfai B, Kuthi L, Varga L, Laczó I, Révész J, et al. Mint: The colorful palette of neuroendocrine neoplasms in the genitourinary tract. Anticancer Research. 2018;**38**(6):3243-3254. DOI: 10.21873/anticanres.12589

[14] Black AJ, Black PC. Mint: Variant histology in bladder cancer: Diagnostic and clinical implications. Translational Cancer Research. 2020;**9**(10):6565-6575. DOI: 10.21037/tcr-20-2169

[15] Mascolo M, Altieri V, Mignogna C, Napodano G, De Rosa G, et al. Mint: Calcitonin-producing well-differentiated neuroendocrine carcinoma (carcinoid tumor) of the urinary bladder: Case report. BMC Cancer. 2005;**5**:88. DOI: 10.1186/1471-2407-5-88

[16] Li H, Xie J, Chen Z, Yang S, Lai Y. Mint: Diagnosis and treatment of a rare tumor-bladder paraganglioma. Molecular and Clinical Oncology. 2020;**13**(4):40. DOI: 10.3892/mco.2020.2110

[17] Hermi A, Ichaoui H, Kacem A, Hedhli H, Gargouri F, et al. Mint: Functional bladder paraganglioma treated by partial cystectomy. Case Reports in Urology. 2019;**2019**:4549790. Published 2019 Nov 12. DOI: 10.1155/2019/4549790

[18] Ranaweera M, Chung E. Mint: Bladder paraganglioma: A report of case series and critical review of current literature. World Journal of Clinical Cases. 2014;**2**(10):591-595. DOI: 10.12998/wjcc.v2.i10.591

[19] Galgano SJ, Porter KK, Burgan C, Rais-Bahrami S. Mint: The role of imaging in bladder cancer diagnosis and staging. Diagnostics (Basel). 2020;**10**(9):703. DOI: 10.3390/diagnostics10090703

[20] Abouelkheir RT, Abdelhamid A, Abou El-Ghar M, El-Diasty T. Mint: Imaging of bladder cancer: Standard applications and future trends. Medicina (Kaunas, Lithuania). 2021;**57**(3):220. Published 2021 Mar 1. DOI: 10.3390/medicina57030220

[21] Moretto P, Wood L, Emmenegger U, Blais N, Mukherjee SD, et al. Mint: Management of small cell carcinoma of the bladder: Consensus guidelines from the Canadian Association of Genitourinary Medical Oncologists (CAGMO). Canadian Urological Association Journal. 2013;**7**(1-2): E44-E56. DOI: 10.5489/cuaj.220

[22] Wängberg B, Nilsson O, Johanson VV, Kölby L, Forssell-Aronsson E, et al. Mint: Somatostatin receptors in the diagnosis and therapy of neuroendocrine tumor. The Oncologist. 1997;**2**(1):50-58 PMID: 10388029

[23] Oronsky B, Ma PC, Morgensztern D, Carter CA. Mint: Nothing but NET: A review of neuroendocrine tumors and carcinomas. Neoplasia. 2017;**19**(12):991-1002. DOI: 10.1016/j.neo.2017.09.002

[24] Tsoli M, Chatzellis E, Koumarianou A, Kolomodi D, Kaltsas G. Mint: Current best practice in the management of neuroendocrine tumors. Therapeutic Advances in Endocrinology and Metabolism. 2018;**10**:2042018818804698. DOI: 10.1177/2042018818804698

[25] Lamberti G, Brizzi MP, Pusceddu S, Gelsomino F, Di Meglio G, et al. Mint: Perioperative chemotherapy in poorly differentiated neuroendocrine neoplasia of the bladder: A multicenter analysis. Journal of Clinical Medicine.

2020;**9**(5):1351. DOI: 10.3390/jcm9051351

[26] Prelaj A, Rebuzzi SE, Magliocca FM, Speranza I, Corongiu E, et al. Mint: Neoadjuvant chemotherapy in neuroendocrine bladder cancer: A case report. American Journal of Case Reports. 2016;**17**:248-253. DOI: 10.12659/ajcr.896989

[27] Pini GM, Uccella S, Corinti M, Colecchia M, Pelosi G, et al. Mint: Primary MiNEN of the urinary bladder: An hitherto undescribed entity composed of large cell neuroendocrine carcinoma and adenocarcinoma with a distinct clinical behavior: Description of a case and review of the pertinent literature. Virchows Archiv. 2021;**479**(1):69-78. DOI: 10.1007/s00428-021-03023-7

[28] Tiong FL. Mint: Long surviving patient with metastatic neuroendocrine bladder cancer: About a case report. Journal of Clinical Case Reports. 2015;**5**:586. DOI: 10.4172/2165-7920.1000586

[29] Zaouit M, Marnissi F, Jouhadi H, Benchekroun N, Elkbi A, et al. Mint: Bladder neuroendocrine carcinoma: About five cases and review of the literature. International Journal of Oncology Research. 2022;**5**:036. DOI: 10.23937/2643-4563/1710036

[30] Hatayama T, Hayashi T, Matsuzaki S, Masumoto H, Yanai H, et al. Mint: Successful treatment of recurrent small cell carcinoma of urinary bladder with pembrolizumab. IJU Case Reports. 2020;**3**(6):252-256. DOI: 10.1002/iju5.12208

[31] Nguyen OTD, Sundstrøm SH, Westvik GS, Røttereng AKS, Melhus MR, et al. Mint: Major durable response of pembrolizumab in chemotherapy refractory small cell bladder cancer: A case report. Case Reports in Oncology. 2020;**13**(3):1059-1066. DOI: 10.1159/000509747

[32] Miller NJ, Khaki AR, Diamantopoulos LN, Bilen MA, Santos V, et al. Mint: Histological subtypes and response to PD-1/PD-L1 blockade in advanced urothelial cancer: A retrospective study. The Journal of Urology. 2020;**204**(1):63-70. DOI: 10.1097/JU.0000000000000761

[33] Looney AM, Nawaz K, Webster RM. Mint: Tumour-agnostic therapies. Nature Reviews. Drug Discovery. 2020;**19**(6):383-384. DOI: 10.1038/d41573-020-00015-1

[34] Lemery S, Fashoyin-Aje L, Marcus L, Casak S, Schneider J, et al. Mint: Development of tissue-agnostic treatments for patients with cancer. Annual Review of Cancer Biology. 2022;**6**(1):147-165. DOI: 10.1146/annurev-cancerbio-060921-021828

[35] European Medicines Agency. KEYTRUDA 25 mg/mL concentrate for solution for infusion. Summary of Product Characteristic. https://www.ema.europa.eu/en/documents/product-information/keytruda-epar-product-information_en.pdf. [Accessed: 2022-06-01]

[36] U. S. Food and Drug Administration. KEYTRUDA® (pembrolizumab) injection, for intravenous use. Highlights of Prescribing Information. https://www.accessdata.fda.gov/drugsatfda_docs/label/2021/125514s096lbl.pdf. [Accessed: 2022-06-01]

[37] European Medicines Agency. VITRAKVI 25 mg hard capsules. VITRAKVI 100 mg hard capsules. Summary of Product Characteristic. https://www.ema.europa.eu/en/

documents/product-information/vitrakvi-epar-product-information_en.pdf. [Accessed: 2022-06-01]

[38] U. S. Food and Drug Administration. VITRAKVI® (larotrectinib) capsules, for oral use. VITRAKVI® (larotrectinib) oral solution. Highlights of Prescribing Information. https://www.accessdata.fda.gov/drugsatfda_docs/label/2021/211710s004lbl.pdf. [Accessed: 2022-06-01]

[39] European Medicines Agency. Rozlytrek 100 mg hard capsules. Rozlytrek 200 mg hard capsules. Summary of Product Characteristic. https://www.ema.europa.eu/en/documents/product-information/rozlytrek-epar-product-information_en.pdf. [Accessed: 2022-06-01]

[40] U. S. Food and Drug Administration. ROZLYTREK (entrectinib) capsules, for oral use. Highlights of Prescribing Information. https://www.accessdata.fda.gov/drugsatfda_docs/label/2019/212725s000lbl.pdf. [Accessed: 2022 06 01]

[41] Gainor JF, Shaw AT. Mint: Novel targets in non-small cell lung cancer: ROS1 and RET fusions. The Oncologist. 2013;**18**(7):865-875. DOI: 10.1634/theoncologist.2013-0095

[42] Almquist D, Ernani V. Mint: The road less traveled: A guide to metastatic ROS1-rearranged non-small-cell lung cancer. Journal of Oncology Practice. 2021;**17**(1):7-14. DOI: 10.1200/OP.20.00819

[43] World Health Organization. Palliative care. Source: WHO. Palliative Care. Facts sheet. [Internet] https://www.who.int/health-topics/palliative-care. [Accessed: 2022-06-01]

[44] Hoerger M, Wayser GR, Schwing G, Suzuki A, Perry LM. Mint: Impact of interdisciplinary outpatient specialty palliative care on survival and quality of life in adults with advanced cancer: A meta-analysis of randomized controlled trials. Annals of Behavioral Medicine. 2019;**53**(7):674-685. DOI: 10.1093/abm/kay077

[45] Hugar LA, Lopa SH, Yabes JG, Yu JA, Turner RM 2nd, et al. Mint: Palliative care use amongst patients with bladder cancer. BJU International. 2019;**123**(6):968-975. DOI: 10.1111/bju.14708

[46] Rades D, Manig L, Janssen S, Schild SE. Mint: A survival score for patients assigned to palliative radiotherapy for metastatic bladder cancer. Anticancer Research. 2017;**37**(3):1481-1484. DOI: 10.21873/anticanres.11473

[47] Robinson AG, Wei X, Mackillop WJ, Peng Y, Booth CM. Mint: Use of palliative chemotherapy for advanced bladder cancer: Patterns of care in routine clinical practice. Journal of the National Comprehensive Cancer Network. 2016;**14**(3):291-298. DOI: 10.6004/jnccn.2016.0034

Chapter 6

Estimation of Some Plant Extract Activity against Bacterial Cystitis Isolated from Urinary Tract Infection

AzalA Al-Rubaeaee, Zahraa Ch. Hameed and Sara Al-Tamemi

Abstract

In this study, 60 urine samples were collected from patients with urinary tract infections who were admitted to Al-Hussein Teaching Hospital between December and February of 2018–2019. A urine sample was collected for culture and crystal formation. Only 57 (95 percent) of the 60 samples on culture were isolated from urinary tract infections caused by various causes. According to the results of the isolation and laboratory diagnosis, as well as biochemical tests, *Staphylococcus saprophyticus*, *Streptococcus agalactiae*, *Escherichia coli*, Klebsiella pneumonia, proteus spp., Morganella morgani, and Pseudomonas aueroginosa were identified in this study. *S. saprophyticus* is the ore predominant in UTIs infection While *Morganella morganii* is the least common result, 8% of the total The isolates are varied in their ability to produce urease enzyme and stone (cast) they were varied in their hemolytic activity. Isolates that able to produce urease in different level which provided as main step in pathogenesis in urinary tract infections and cast formation, Zea mays, curcumine and canberry were shown very high effectively to inhibit stone in the percent of (11–13), respectively coffee and Ziziphus gave results varied in their activity.

Keywords: UTIS, cystitis, *M.morganii*, plant extract, bacterial cystitis

1. Introduction

Urease production is regarded as an important virulence factor in bacterial pathogenicity because the ammonia produced by this enzyme raises the pH, which has important medical implications. Urease is a virulence factor found in pathogenic bacteria that cause gastric ulcers, urinary stone formation, pyelonephritis, and other human health issues [1].

Although symptoms can aid in the diagnosis of a UTI, they may not accurately localize the infection within the urinary tract. However, in many cases, urinary tract colonization is asymptomatic. Cystitis (bladder infection) is the most common type of UTI, characterized by irritative symptoms such as urinary urgency, frequency, dysuria, hematuria, foul-smelling urine, and suprapubic pain. In addition to cystitis, these symptoms are also common for urethritis and prostatitis. An associated epididymitis, diagnosed reliably by physical examination in men, is an easily localizable variation of UTI. Symptoms of "upper urinary tract" infections, such as pyelonephritis, may include those associated with cystitis, as well as fever, rigors, flank or abdominal pain, and nausea and vomiting [2]. The aims of our study is evaluation of some plant extract on bladder stone and well done by this objectives:-

1. Isolation the pathogenic bacterial SPP. From urinary tract infections

2. Investigateion bacterial isolates on urease production abbility.

3. In vitro stone foramtion

4. Estimation the activity of some plants on this stone

As a result, the organism has an easily assimilated nitrogen source. Urease promotes virulence in uropathogenic bacteria. As a result, the urinary tract becomes alkaline. Increased urine pH can cause the formation of struvite stones, which contain the infecting organism, increased attachment of bacteria to the renal epithelium, direct renal tissue damage, and the activation of certain antibiotics [3].

Because urinary stones are a mixture of compounds de-posited as a result of metabolic disorders and infections, their chemical composition is not uniform. The fact that urolithiasis promotes the development of infections, and bacteria easily colonize porous stone surfaces, may explain the diverse composition of the stones [4].

Struvite stones are also referred to as 'infection stones' and 'triple phosphate stones'. Struvite stone formation can only be sustained if ammonia production is increased and the urine pH is raised to reduce phosphate solubility. Only when urine is infected with a urease-producing organism, such as Proteus, can both of these requirements be met. Urease degrades urea to produce ammonia and carbon dioxide: 2NH3 + CO2 = Urea With a pK of 9.0, the ammonia/ammonium buffer pair produces highly alkaline urine rich in ammonia. Urease is an enzyme that breaks down urea into ammonia and carbonic acid.

alkaline urine rich in ammonia. Urease splits urea into ammonia and carbonic acid:

$$\mathrm{NH2} - \mathrm{CO} - \mathrm{NH2} \rightarrow H2\mathrm{CO3} + 2\ \mathrm{NH3} \tag{1}$$

Ammonia then mixes with water to produce ammonium hydroxide and under these alkaline conditions, carbonic acid moves toward bicarbonate and carbonate ions.

$$\mathrm{NH_3} + 2\,H_2O \rightarrow 2\ \mathrm{NH_4}^+ + 2\ \mathrm{oh}^- \tag{2}$$

Thus, the alkalinisation of urine by the urease reaction causes the formation of NH_4^+, which favors the formation of carbonate ions (CO_3^{2-}) and trivalent phosphate ions (PO_4^{3-}). This in turn causes struvite and carbonate apatite formation (Sun *et al.*, 2010).

$$\mathrm{CO_3}^{2-} + 10\ \mathrm{Ca}^{2+} + 6\ \mathrm{PO_4}^{3-} \rightarrow \mathrm{Ca_{10}}\ (\mathrm{PO_4})_6\mathrm{CO_3} \tag{3}$$

$$6\,H_2O + Mg^{2+} + NH_4{}^{+} + PO_4{}^{3-} \rightarrow MgNH_4PO_46H_2O \qquad (4)$$

These components all play different roles in the plant, resulting in a variety of potential health benefits from their consumption. Microorganisms have developed resistance to various antibiotics that are currently in use, as is well known in the medical field. This phenomenon has caused enormous clinical issues in the treatment of diseases caused by such microorganisms.

It appears to be a urease inhibitor with a mechanism. Plants have a natural polyphenol structure that consists of two o-methoxy phenols attached symmetrically through a, −unsaturated -diketone linker that also induces keto-enol tautomerism. It is possible that this compound inhibits urease activity via a chelate interaction that binds to the urease active site; as a result, some plant extracts form a stable complex with urease and, as a result, the enzyme is inhibited.

Proteus is a Gram-negative, rod-shaped bacteria, non-spore forming and facultative anaerobic, catalase positive, oxidase negative and non- lactose fermenter. It belongs to the family Enterobacteriaceae [5].

The first description of *Proteus* bacteria was made in 1885 by Hauser, who named them after the character in Homer's Odyssey who 'has the power of assuming different shapes to escape being questioned' (Wang and Pan, 2014). There are currently four recognized species of *Proteus*: *P. mirabilis*, *Proteus penneri*, *P. vulgaris*, and *Proteus myxofaciens* [6].

This bacterium has to measure (1–3) μm in length and (0.4–0.8) μm in diameter, motile by peritrichous flagella, chemo-organotrophic, made a respiratory and a fermentative type of metabolism not require oxygen, so it called facultative anaerobic [7], made pale colonies shape when growing on MacConkey and when grown on blood agar (that causes β hemolysis on blood agar) with distinct fishy odor. Also, it made rings of swarming motility in an agar media [8].

Morganella morganii:- Morganii and M. sibonii are Gram-negative bacilli that belong to the tribe Proteae of the family Enterobacteriaceae. It is naturally present in the environment and in the intestinal tracts of humans, mammals, and reptiles. Despite its widespread distribution, it is an uncommon cause of human infections [9].

M. morganii was first identified as a cause of urinary tract infections in the late 1930s, and only a few reports of infections due to this pathogen have been published since then. It is most common in postoperative patients and is mostly associated with urinary tract infections. Bacteremia/sepsis in both children and adults Skin and soft tissue infections, meningitis, ecthyma, and endophthalmitis [10].

The genus Zizyphus belongs to the Rhamnaceae family. It is a genus of about 100 species of deciduous or evergreen trees and shrubs found in tropical and subtropical regions. PACs have recently received a lot of attention due to the health benefits that they have been linked to [11].

Cranberries are composed of 88% water and a mixture of organic acids, vitamin C, flavonoids, anthocyanidins, proanthocyanidins (PACs), catechins, and triterpinoids [12].

Curcumin (diferuloylmethane, chemical formula: $C_{21}H_{20}O_6$ is a yellow-orange pigment extracted from the roots of turmeric (*Curcuma longa*). It usually exists in two tautomeric forms: keto and enol, The enol form has a higher energy stability. Curcumin has gained popularity due to its diverse biological activities. Turmeric gained popularity in the 1970s after it was discovered to have anti-inflammatory properties [12].

The significance of turmeric in medicine has changed since the antioxidant properties of other plants were discovered, therefore, it is found thatplants possesses antitumour, antibacterial, antifungal and antiviral properties additionally, these plant does not exhibit toxicity to either animal or humans even at high doses, the case of struvite crystallization induced by bacteria in relation to urinary stone formation. Urease inhibitors bind to it and inhibit its activity by preventing the hydrolysis of urea to ammonia and carbon dioxide. There are two types of urease inhibitors: I mechanism-based directed mode; (ii) active-site directed mode The active-site directed inhibitors resemble urea, the enzyme's substrate, in structure. Mechanism-based directed inhibitors interfere with the catalysis mechanism of the enzyme, causing it to be inhibited or inactivated [13].

It appears to be a mechanism-based urease inhibitor. Plants have a chemical structure that consists of two o-methoxy phenols attached symmetrically via a, −unsaturated -diketone linker, which also induces keto-enol tautomerism, making it a natural polyphenol. It is possible that this compound inhibits urease activity via a chelate interaction, which binds to the urease active site; as a result, some plant extracts form a stable complex with urease, inhibiting urease activity. The diketone moiety of plants has chelating properties toward transition metals, including nickel. Curcumin chelation toward transition metals such as iron and copper has been found to be beneficial in the treatment of Alzheimer's disease [14].

2. Materials

2.1 Specimens

A total of 60 urine samples were collected from patients admitted to Al-Hussein teaching Hospital, during a period extending from September 2018 to December 2018.

Urine samples were collected in sterile cups, as all patients had signs and symptoms of UTI and they were diagnosed as having UTI by the Urologists.

3. Methods

3.1 Preparation of reagents and solutions

3.1.1 Reagents

3.1.1.1 Catalase reagent

This reagent was used with a concentration of 3%. It was prepared by adding H2O2 to D.W. (v/v). It was used for identification of catalase producing bacteria by looking for appearance of air bubbles which indicate positivity.

3.1.1.2 Oxidase reagent

This reagent was prepared freshly, by dissolving 1gm of (tetramethyl-paraphenylene-diamine-dihydrochloride) in 100 ml of D.W. and kept in a dark bottle. It immediately used for the identification of bacteria positive for oxidase production by the appearance of dark purple color as a positive result.

3.1.1.3 Methyl red reagent

Methyl red reagent is prepared by dissolving 0.1 gm of methyl red in 300 ml of (95%) ethanol and then the volume is completed to 500 ml by D.W. It is used to identify the complete glucose hydrolysis.

3.1.1.4 Coagulase test

It is an important method for detection of ability to produce coagulase and differentiation between coagulase-producing and non-producing staphylococci. Bacterial broth was added to fresh plasma, and incubated at 37°C and examined after 1,2,3 and 4 hours. The test was read by tilting the tube and observing for clot formation in the plasma.

4. Preparation of culture media

A group of culture media were prepared according to the instructions of the manufactures company and sterilized by autoclaving at 121°C for 15 minutes.

4.1 Blood agar medium

Blood agar medium was prepared by dissolving blood agar base in distal water. It was autoclaved cooled to 50°C. 5% fresh human blood was added and mixed well. This medium was used to cultivate bacterial isolates and to determine the ability of bacteria to hemolyse blood cell.

4.2 Mannitol-salt agar medium

Mannitol salt agar was prepared according to manufacturer. It was used to detect ability to ferment mannitol.

4.3 Nutrient agar medium

Nutrient agar medium was prepared according to the manufacturing company. It was used for general experiments, cultivation and activation of bacterial isolates when it is necessary.

4.4 Nutrient broth

This medium was used to grow and preserve the bacterial isolates. Nutrient broth medium was prepared according to the method suggested by the manufacturing company.

4.5 Urea agar medium

Urea agar medium was prepared by adding 10 ml of urea solution (20% sterilized by Millipore filter paper) in volume of autoclaved urea agar base and completed up to 100 ml distilled water and cooled to 50°C, the pH was adjusted to 7.1. then medium was put into test tubes and allowed to solidify in a slant form. It was used to test ability of bacteria to produce urease enzyme.

4.6 Brain heart infusion broth

Brain-heart infusion broth was prepared according to the manufacturing company. It was used for detection of different biochemical tests.

4.7 MacConkey agar medium

MacConkey agar medium was prepared according to the method recommended by the manufacturing company. It was used for the primary isolation of most Gram-negative bacteria and to differentiate lactose fermenters from non-lactose fermenters.

4.8 Brain heart infusion (BHI) broth: glycerol medium

This medium was prepared by mixing 5 ml of glycerol with 95 ml of BHI broth (sterilized by autoclave). It was used for preservation of bacterial isolates as stock for long time.

4.9 Simmon-citrate medium

Simmon-citrate medium is prepared according to the manufacturing company. It has been used for determining the ability of bacteria to utilize citrate as the sole source of carbon.

4.10 Kligler iron agar medium

Kligler-Iron agar was used for determining glucose and lactose fermentation and possible hydrogen sulfide (H2S) production as a first step in the identification of Gram-ve bacilli.

4.11 Motility medium

It was prepared by dissolving 0.5 gm of agar-agar in 100 ml of brain-heart infusion broth and autoclaved, then the contents were dispensed into test tube.

5. Collection of specimens

Urine specimens were collected under aseptic procedure, to avoid any possible contamination. 10 ml of mid-stream urine samples are collected from patients suffering from UTIs, urine samples are collected in sterile screw-cap containers. Each specimen is immediately inoculated onto the blood agar plates and MacConkey's plates. All plates are incubated at 37°C for 24 hrs.

6. Laboratory diagnosis

According to the diagnostic procedures recommended, The isolation and identification of Staphylococci species in specimens are performed as follows:

6.1 Colonial morphology and microscopic examination

6.1.1 Colonial morphology

All specimens were cultivated on blood agar, Nutrient and MacConkey agar media by swabbing and incubated at 37°C for 18-24 hrs.Each primary positive culture is identified depending on the phenotypic properties such as (colony size, shape, color and nature of pigments, translucency, edge, elevation, and texture).

6.1.2 Microscopic examination

The morphology of bacterial cells is investigated by Gram-stain to observe shape, arrangement of cells and type of reaction by using Gram-stain. Then, specific biochemical tests are done for each isolates for the final identification.

6.1.3 Motility test

After preparation of semisolid media, the bacterial colonies were inoculated by stabbing-down to the center of the tube to about half the depth of the medium. The cultured tubes were incubated at 37°C and were examined after 6 hours, 1 and 2 days. Non-motile bacteria had generally restricted to the stab line and given sharply defined margins with leaving the surrounding medium clearly transparent, while motile bacteria give diffuse hazy growth that spread throughout the medium rendering it slightly opaque.

6.2 Biochemical tests

The following biochemical tests are performed for the identification of Staphylococcus species isolates:

6.2.1 Coagulase test

Method of Benson (2001), include several colonies of bacterial growth were transferred with a loop to a tube containing 5 ml of Nutrient broth. The tube was covered to prevent evaporation and incubated at 37°C in the incubator over-night. After incubation, tube mixed and centrifuged, 0.5 ml of the supernatant withdrawn and mixed with 0.5 ml of fresh human plasma, then incubated in the water bath at 37°C for several hours.

If the plasma is coagulated, the organism is coagulase-positive. Some coagulations occurred in 30 minutes or several hours later. Any degree of coagulation, from a loose clot suspended in plasma to a solid clot, was considered to be a positive result, even if it takes 24 hours to occur.

6.2.2 Catalase test

Transferring the bacterial growth by wood stick and put it on the surface of a clean slide and add a drop of (3% H2O2), positive result when the gas bubbles appear.

6.2.3 Oxidase test

Filter paper is soaked with a freshly made reagent, and the colony to be tested is taken up with a sterile wooden stick and put over the filter paper. A positive result is indicated by a deep purple color which appeared within 5–10 seconds.

6.2.4 Citrate utilization test

The surface of simmons citrate slant medium is inoculated with the colony of tested bacteria and incubated at 37°C 18-24 hrs. Conversion of the indicator's color from green to blue indicates that the organism was able to utilize citrate as a sole source of carbon.

6.2.5 Methyl red test

Tubes of MR-VP broth are seeded with the selected bacterial colonies and incubated at 37°C for 48 hrs. Then 5 drops of methyl red reagent are added to it, the appearance and observation of red color means a positive result and a complete analysis of glucose.

6.2.6 Mannitol fermentation test

Mannitol Salt Agar was inoculated with bacterial colonies then incubated at 37C° for 24 hours. The color changed from pink to bright yellow as the bacteria was lactose fermenter, or unchanging color of the medium was a negative result.

6.3 Virulence factors test

6.3.1 Urease test

This test was done by inoculating the prepared urea medium with bacterial growth. The tubes were incubated for 24–48 hours at 37°C. The change of color medium into pink indicated a positive result.

6.3.2 Haemolysin production on blood agar

Detection of hemolysin production was carried out by inoculating a blood agar with bacterial isolates, then incubated at 37°C for 24 hrs. The appearance of a clear zone around the colonies indicated a complete hemolysis (ß- hemolysis) while greenish zone around the colonies referred to partial hemolysis (α- hemolysis), no change in the medium referred to no hemolysis (γ- hemolysis).

6.4 In vitro stone formation

A fresh urine sample was obtained from a healthy control with no history of urinary stones or urogenital infectious diseases. It was sterilized by filtration. Ability to forma stone was detected by growing bacterial species aerobically at 37°C for 24 hours in brain heart infusion broth which was enriched with 1% Tween 80 and 10% serum. 1 ml of 1: 10 dilution in human urine of an overnight culture of bacteria was inoculated in to 9 ml of the sterile urine.

E. coli (known to be non-urease-producer) was inoculated in the same mentioned above.

All inoculums gave a final count of about 107 CFU/ml.

A control of 10 ml of urine (from the same person) was also studied.

All tubes were incubated at the same incubation conditions (at 37°Cfor overnight).

Ammonium concentration (indophenol method; appendix), turbidity and pH were determined at the beginning of experiment and after 4, 8 and 24 hours of incubation.

Sediment was examined at the same intervals and crystals, if any, were identified both macro- and microscopically.

The inhibition factor were added.

6.5 Plant extract preparation

50 gm of the powdered of each samples (curcumine, Zea mays, Ziziphus, coffee) dissolved in 500 ml of distilled water the final concentration of each plant extract is 50 gm/ml while the cranberry were used as a template with its exact concentration.

7. Results and discussion

7.1 Isolation and identification bacterial urinary tract infections

7.1.1 Isolation of species

A total of 60 urine samples were obtained from patients suffering from urinary tract infection who are admitted to Al-Hussein Teaching Hospital, at the period from December to February 2018–2019. Among 60 clinical samples, only 57 showed positive results, as shown in **Table 1**.

In this study, Staphylococcus *saprophyticus*, *Streptococcus agalactiae, Escherichia coli, Klebsiella pneumonia, proteus spp., Morganella morgani* and *Pseudomonas aueroginosa* that were isolated and identified in this study, as shown in **Table 2** and the **Figure 1** Show the distribution rate of isolation.

No. of urine samples	No. of culture	
	No. of negative culture	No. of positive culture
60 samples	3(5%)	57(95%)

Table 1.
Number and percentage of bacteria isolated from urine samples of patients with urinary tract infections.

Bacterial spp.	No. of isolation			%
	Male	Female	Total	
Klebsiella	2	5	7	12%
Staphylococcus saprophyticus	—	12	12	21%
Proteus	6	4	10	19%
Morganella morgani	2	3	5	8%
Pseudomonas aueroginosa	5	3	8	14%
E.coli	4	5	9	16%
Streptococcus agalactiae	—	6	6	10%
Total	19 (34%)	38(66%)	57	100%

Table 2.
Prevalence and distribution of bacterial pathogens according to gender of patients.

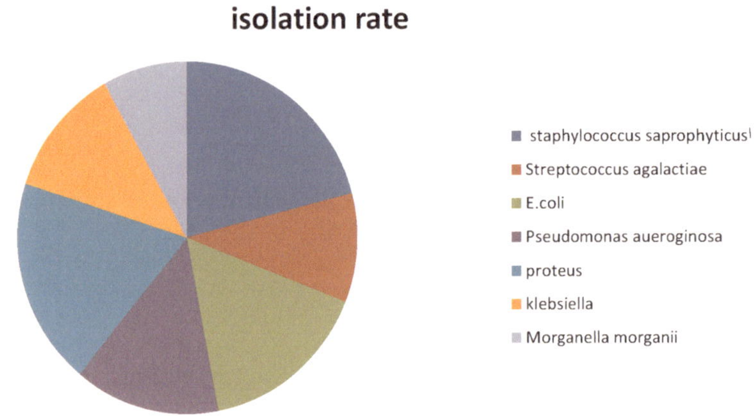

Figure 1.
Distribution of bacterial Spp. isolation rate.

It was observed that *Klebsiella pneumoniae* is rods, catalase positive, oxidase negative and hemolysin producer, non-motile, lactose fermenter on MacConkey agar, the colonies appear pink to red in color, with mucoid phenotype.

Besides, the isolates were urease and capsule producers, having positive results for vogues proskaur and negative for methyl red and H_2S production test. All the isolates of *klebsiella pneumoniae* were fermenter for glucose, lactose sucrose, L-arabinose, D-mannitol and maltos.

Regarding, *Staphylococcus saprophyticus*, this bacteria is isolated only from women patients with UTI at a rate 21%. This bacteria is highly prevalence among young women, and also is considered pathogen in UTI. Many studies indicate that *S. saprophyticus* can cause UTI in young females and considered as the second causes of UTI among this age group (below 15 years old) after *E. coli* [15–17].

Streptococcus agalactiae (group B *Streptococcus*) is a major cause of neonatal infectious disease in humans in many countries and is carried asymptomatically by a large proportion of adults. It is also recognized as an emerging pathogen in human adults [18].

GBS is also an important cause of morbidity and mortality in the elderly and in immuno-compromised adults. Primary manifestations of adult GBS disease include bacteremia, skin and soft tissue infections, pneumonia, osteomyelitis and urinar y tract infections [19, 20].

According to [21] only (16.7%) of urine samples were obtained from patients with suspected UTI were positive from coagulase negative staphylococcus, and this result is lesser than that obtained in this study, Isolation rate of *Proteus spp*. Similar to [22] who found that percentage 7(7%) of *Proteus*. The variation in bacterial isolation between studies may be attributed to many factors such as sanitary practices in hospitals and staff, environmental conditions, isolation and identification techniques, social and cultural level of patients, and use multidrug (antibiotics) that may lead to developing in bacterial resistance ability, or may be due to differences in the size of samples; all these factors may employ together and play an important role in inhibit or stimulate the growth and distribution of pathogenic bacteria in hospitals.

7.2 Identification of bacterial *spp*

The identification of any bacteria depends mainly on the cultural, biochemical characteristics and microscopic patterns. These organisms varying from cocci to (bacilli) rods microscopically searching on is motile or not, spore forming, coagulase and catalase.

Most *Staphylococcus*; on blood agar, the colonies tend to be non-pigmented, smooth, entire, glistening, and opaque colonies, However, the isolates were shown to be catalase positive, oxidase negative, coagulase negative, and mannitol fermentation negative. Also, all isolates were non-motile and negative for each starch hydrolysis, gelatin hydrolysis, methyl red and citrate utilization test.

The identification of *Proteus* is Gram- negative bacilli, catalase positive,have white colony with fushy oder and showe swarming motality. *M. morganii* can produce the enzyme catalase, so is able to convert hydrogen peroxide to water and oxygen. This is a common enzyme found in most living organisms. In addition, it is indole test-positive representing this organism can split tryptophan to indole, pyruvate, and ammonia. Methyl redtests positive in Morganella morganii, an indicator dye that turns red in acidic solutions. is facultatively anaerobic and oxidase-negative. Its colonies appear off-white and opaque in color, when grown on blood agar plates. It is straight rods, about 0.6–0.7 μm in diameter and 1.0–1.7 μm in length.

8. Complicated and simple urinary tract infections

A total (57) isolates of bacteria 33 (18.66%) isolated obtained from patient with complicated urinary tract infection and a 24 (39.2%) isolated obtained from patients with simple urinary tract infection from both sex as shown in **Table 3**, While the **Figure 2** shows the comparison between them.

No. of *bacterial* Isolated	Complicated UTIs	simple UTIs
57	33(57.8%)	24(42.1%)

Table 3.
Bacterial isolated from complicated and simple urinary tract infections.

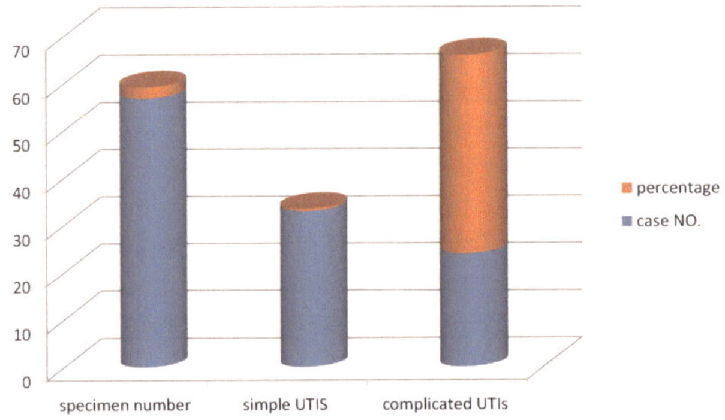

Figure 2.
Show the comparison between complicated and simple UTIs.

Cause of UTI	No. of patients
Renal stone	20
Nephrostomy	1
JJ stent	1
Bladder stone	1
Chronic pyelonephritis	1
Ca. of bladder	2
Urethral tumor	1
BPH	3
Immune compromised, leukemia	2
Urethral stricture	1

Table 4.
Patient with complicated urinary tract infection.

In the case of complicated UTI which includes several cases shown in **Table 4**.

Complicated urinary infection occurs in both women and men, and in any age group. Because uncomplicated urinary infection is rare in men, any male urinary infection is usually considered complicated (**Figure 3**) [23].

Recurrent urinary infection in postmenopausal women is associated with genetic and behavioral risk factors similar to those seen in younger women with acute uncomplicated urinary infection, such as a higher likelihood of being a no secretor and a history of prior urinary infection [24].

However, postmenopausal women with recurrent urinary infection are also more likely to have increased residual urine volume, cystoceles and prior genitourinary

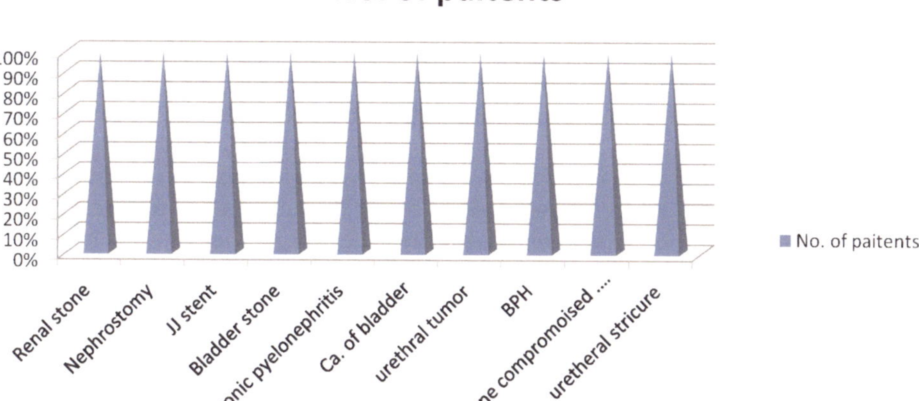

Figure 3.
Distribution of complicated UTI cases.

surgery than are women without infection, and these associations are consistent with complicated infection. Thus, as a population, postmenopausal women with recurrent urinary infection encompass elements consistent with both uncomplicated and complicated urinary infection.

In case of complicated UTI, the result of this study was agreement with results obtained by [25] who found that these bacteria found in complicated UTI with percentage (60.8%). This result was dis- agreement with the result obtained by [26] as they found that the percentage of isolated percentage.

Also, the result in this study is closed to that obtained by [27] who found that percentage 44% from complicated UTI, and the results obtained by [28] that they were isolated bacterial *spp.* from renal calculi in percentage 21% was not agreement with results in this study.

On the other hand, the case of simple UTI with includes seven isolated from woman, including four pregnant women, two males from the other nine samples.

9. *In vitro* struvite stone formation by bacterial spp.

Struvite stones are thought to develop in urinary tract infected with urea splitting bacteria; the bacterial urease hydrolyzes urea, leading to hyperammonuria and alkalinization of urine with consequent crystallization of struvite.

In the present study, the stone forming ability of urease positive isolates investigated through an experiment testing the pH and crystals of human urine inoculated with, *E. coli* as a control and controlled urine with no bacteria at 0, 4, 8, and 24 hours of incubation.

When human urine was inoculated with bacteria a gradual increase in the cell density was noticed until the 4th hour when the rate of proliferation became faster, increasing the microbial population to the maximum when examined after an overnight incubation, during the experimental bacterial growth in human urine, the primary urine pH, and crystals were measure, and re-measured again at 4, 8 and 24 hours of incubation. At the onset of the experiment, the urine pH was about (5.5). When isolates grew in human urine, there was a slight elevation in the urine pH at the first

4 hours, reaching about (6.2), at 8 hours reach to (7.5) and maximized after 24 hours up to (9). However, this is not the case when *E. coli* grew at the same experimental conditions, as it was expected, there was a very minor elevation in the pH, whereas, the final reading was 6.0. On the other hand there were no changes in the pH of control urine which was free of bacteria during the period of study. The results were shown in **Figure 4**.

Struvite stones formation associated with urinary infection by urease production isolates are thought to be as a consequence of hyper ammonuria and alkalinization of urine associated with this bacterium growth [29].

The numbers of crystals seen microscopically increased gradually parallel with that of both the pH, reaching a maximum number after 24 hours of incubation when white sediment appeared at the bottom of the tube at that time (**Table 5**).

However, as it was expected *E. coli* growth resulted in no increase in the number of crystals seen microscopically as in the case of other non-urease producer organisms, and urine inoculated with no bacteria did not alter the number of crystals at all (**Figure 5**). There was no sediment observed in case of both *E coli pseudomonas* the control urine after an overnight incubation (**Figure 6**).

P. merabilis is a relatively fastidious microorganism and is probably less virulent than other gram negative bacilli usually involved in urinary tract infection, urease enzyme produced by this bacterium plays a major role in the pathogenesis of struvite

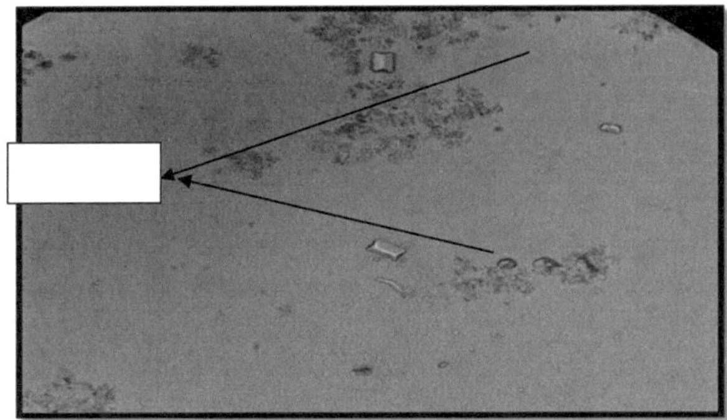

Figure 4.
Stone formation by positive urease, bacteria (40×).

Bacterium	No. of crystals/Hpf microscope at hour			
	zero	4	8	24
Strep. agalactiae	0–4	4–8	8–12	**12–20**
Staph. saprophyticus	0–6	6–8	8–11	12–25
Merothrips morgani	0–6	6–10	10–15	15–20
Klebsiella	0–7	7–10	11–17	12–28
Proteus	0–3	3–8	5–10	20–30
E. coli	0–3	0–3	0–3	0–3
P. aueroginosa	0–2	0–2	0–2	0–2

Table 5.
Number of crystals according to the time in bacterial isolated from complicated and simple urinary tract infection.

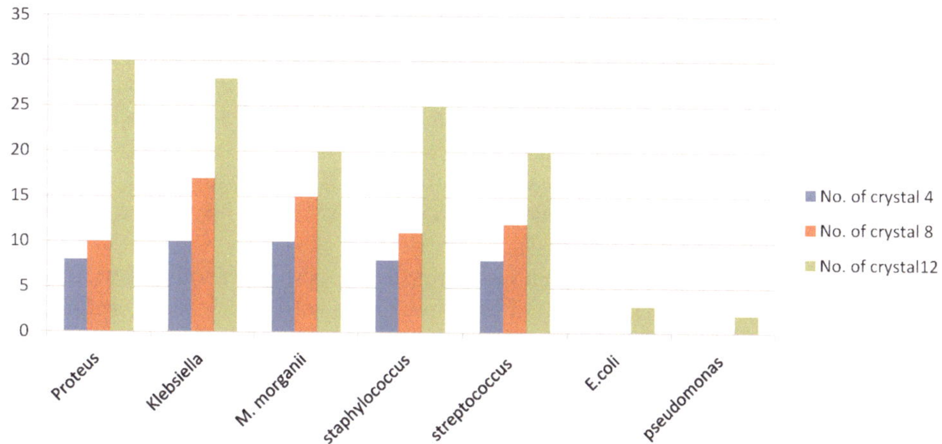

Figure 5.
Shows stone formation according to the time.

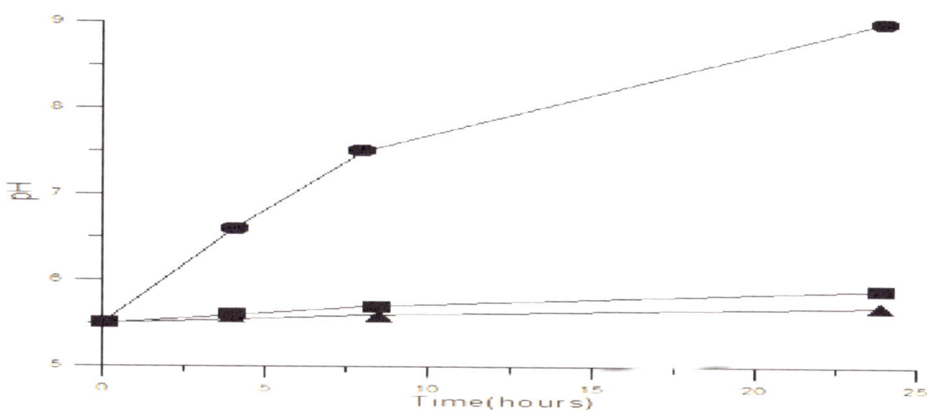

Figure 6.
Stone formation by bacteria with correlation to the time.

stone formation, and it is agreed to be the direct cause of hyperammonuria and alkalinization of urine seen in UTI caused by this bacterium.

Struvite is one of the main components of infectious urinary stones, which are caused by the activity of microorganisms that produce urease, primarily Proteus species. One of the primary causes of urinary stone formation is the aggregation of precipitating particles and bacteria.

10. Effect of some plants extracts on struvite stone formation

The effect of some plant extract on stone formation was investigated; it was found that the activity of curcumin were performed an in vitro experiment of struvite growth from human urine. The results demonstrate that curcumin exhibits the effect against isolates inhibiting the activity of urease—an enzyme produced by these microorganisms. Addition of curcumin decreases the efficiency of growth of struvite compared with the absence of curcumin.

The results show that the urine pH was about (4.5). When bacteria grew in human urine and give a very high rate of stone formation followed by, and added curcumin and crambery, there was a slight elevation in the urine pH at the first 4 hours, reduced increase pH to reaching about (5.5), at 8 hours the pH was reach to (6) and after 24 hours the pH was (7.5) (**Table 6**).

This result was agrrement with result obtained by [30] who found that the experiment of added curcumin has demonstrated that the curcumin a lower concentration has inhibitor urease activity (**Figure 7**).

In the case of addition of curcumin our experiment runs differently. First, the solubility of curcumin in the solution of human urine is relatively low. Therefore, we have initially observed unsolvable particlcs of curcumin, resulting in "stellar" aggregates. Furthermore, individual struvite crystals appear later in the absence of curcumin. Furthermore, the addition of curcumin reduces the size and number of struvite crystals.

No. of cast Bacterial Isolates	Free without inhibition	Plant extract				
		Zea mays	Curcumin	*Cranberry*	*Ziziphus*	Coffee
Proteus	30	19	17	19	22	25
Klebsiella	28	9	11	8	10	12
Morganella morganii	20	8	10	10	11	11
Staphylocuccus	25	9	11	11	18	18
Streptococcus	20	10	10	17	19	20

Table 6.
Effect of plant extract against struvite stone.

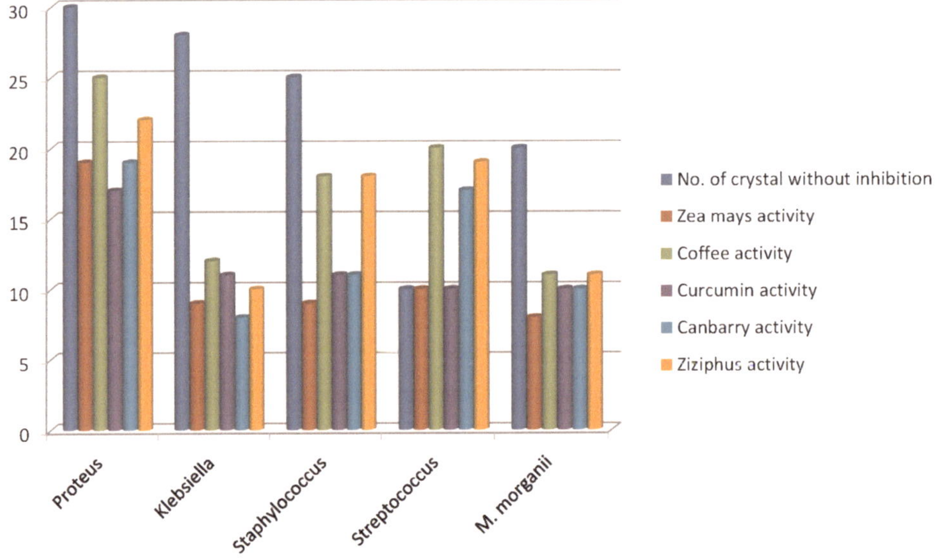

Figure 7.
Shows the plant extract activity against stone.

Struvite crystals form much later when curcumin is present than when it is not. Two factors could contribute to a slower pH increase. For starters, curcumin has the potential to act as a bactericide. Second, while curcumin may inhibit urease activity, it has no effect on the viability of the bacterium. In contrast, curcumin inhibits urease activity.

Curcumin as well as *Zea mays* and *Ziziphus* leave has attracted attention because of its various biological activities. Modern interest in turmeric began in 1970s when it was found that turmeric possesses anti-inflammatory properties. Therefore, plant extracts are widely studied and it is found that curcumin possesses also antitumor, antibacterial, antifungal and antiviral properties, Curcumin is a powerful agent that can be used in a variety of pharmacological applications. Furthermore, curcumin is not toxic to either animals or humans at high doses. Even at doses of 8–10 g/day, curcumin is pharmacologically safe [31]. Tween 80 in culture media promotes the formation of struvite stone by stabilizing urease activity. The current study has confirmed that urease is important in stone formation.

Cranberries are made up of 88 percent water and a variety of organic acids, vitamin C, flavonoids, anthocyanidins, catechins, and triterpinoids. These components all play different roles in the plant, which results in a variety of potential health benefits from their consumption. PACs have recently received a lot of attention due to the health benefits that have been linked to them.

Certain cranberry components have anti-adhesive effects on specific uropathogens. Cranberries contain three types of Mavonoids (Mavonols, anthocyanins, and as well as catechins, hydroxyl cinnamic acid, and other phenolic acids and triterpenoids. Anthocyanins are absorbed and transported through the human circulatory system without causing any chemical changes in the urine.

Therefore, PACs can reduce the bacterial attachment to host tissues and prevent biofilm synthesis. It has been suggested by that disruption of quorum sensing by PACs might be the other reason of decrease in biofilm production. Cranberry can be an effective preventive measure for UTIs as it inhibits adhesion and biofilm formation of uropathogenic bacteria.

11. Conclusion

In this chapter, it is included that.

The prevalence of pathogens in complicated UTI is more than in simple UTI because its virulence as well as its ability to causes diseases.

Staphylococcus saprophyticus are the more predominant pathogen in UTI infection in female at the reproductive age.

Urease enzyme are sole of strutative cystitis.

All urease-producing bacteria are able to cause cystitis.

Successful uses of curcumine, zea mays, chrampry, ziziphus leave and coffee to eradicated the Bacterial cystitis.

Acknowledgements

We want to thanks and appreciation all staff in Al-Husseiny teaching hospital emergency for their cooperation during our research.

Author details

AzalA Al-Rubaeaee*, Zahraa Ch. Hameed and Sara Al-Tamemi
Department of Medical Laboratories Techniques, Al-Safwa University College, Karbala, Iraq

*Address all correspondence to: azal.alaa@alsafwa.edu.iq

References

[1] Adhikari KIP, Mukherjee T. Physicochemical studies on the evaluation of the antioxidant activity of herbal extracts and active principles of m some Indianmedicinal plants. Journal of Clinical Biochemistry and Nutrition. 2007;**40**(3):174-183

[2] Al-Bassam WW, Al-Kazaz A. The isolation and characterization of Proteus mirabilis from different clinical samples. J. Biotech. Res. Cen. 2013;7(2):24-30

[3] Al-Sabari AHR. Isolation and Molecular Characterization of Morganella morganii Isolates from Catheter Associated Urinary Tract Infection [Thesis]. Iraq: College of medicine, Babylon University; 2011

[4] Amtul Z, Rahman AU, Siddiqui RA, Choudhary MI. Chemistry and mechanism of urease inhibition. Microbial Ecology. 2002;**72**(4):741-758

[5] Barbour EK, Hajj ZG, Hamadeh S, Shaib HA, Farran MT, Araj G, et al. Comparison of phenotypic and virulence genes characteristics in human and chicken isolates of Proteus mirabilis. Pathogens and Global Health. 2012; **106**(6):352-357

[6] Burne RA, Chen YY. Bacterial ureases in infectious diseases. Microb. Inf. 2000; **2**(5):533-542

[7] De Fazio A, Thummar H, Rothberg M, Motamedinia P, Badalato G, Gupta M. The modern era struvite stone: Patterns of urinary infection and colonization. Journal of Urology. 2015;**193**(4):e451-e452

[8] Doyle JD, Oldring K, Churchley J, Parsons SA. Struvite formation and the fouling propensity of different materials. Water Research. 2002;**36**(16):3971-3978

[9] Drzewiecka D. Significance and roles of Proteus spp bacteria in natural environments. International Journal of Molecular Sciences. 2016;**16**(6): 12119-12130

[10] Dzutsev A, Trinchieri G. Proteus mirabilis: The enemy within. Immunity. 2015;**42**(4):602-604

[11] Eiff VC, Peters G, Heilmann C. Pathogenesis of infections due to coagulase-negative staphylococci. The Lancet Infectious Diseases. 2002;**2**:677-685

[12] Eydelnant IA, Tufenkji N. Cranberry derived proanthocyanidins reduce bacterial adhesion to selected biomaterials. Langmuir. 2008;**24**(18): 10273-10281

[13] Ferreira AM, Bonesso MF, Mondelli AL, Cunha MLR. Identification of staphylococcus saprophyticus isolated from patients with urinary tract infection using a simple set of biochemical tests correlating with 16S–23S interspace region molecular weight patterns. Journal of Microbiological Methods. 2012;**91**: 406-411

[14] Forbes BA, Daniel FS, Alice SW. Bailey and Scott's Diagnostic Microbiology. 12th ed. USA: Mosby Elsevier Company; 2007

[15] Guay DRP. Cranberry and urinary tract infections. Drugs. 2009;**69**(7): 775-807

[16] Jarallah E, Jawad M. Study of some virulence factors of Proteus mirabilis isolated from urinary stones patients. Journal of Biology, Agriculture and Healthcare. 2015;**5**(32): 85-95

[17] King NP, Beatson SA, Totsika M, Ulett GC, Alm RA, Manning PA, et al. Uaf B is a serine-rich repeat adhesin of staphylococcus saprophyticus that mediates binding to fibronectin, fibrinogen and human uroepithelial cells. Microbiology. 2011;**157**:1161-1175

[18] King NP, Sakinc T, Zakour NL, Totsika M, Heras B, Simerska P, et al. Characterisation of a cell wall-anchored protein of staphylococcus saprophyticus associated with linoleic acid resistance. Microbiology. 2012;**8**(12):1471-2180

[19] Konieczna I, Zarnowiec P, Kwinkowski M, Kolesinska B, Fraczyk J, Kaminski Z, et al. Bacterial urease and its role in long-lasting human diseases. Current Protein & Peptide Science. 2012; **13**(8):789-806

[20] Kurihara Y, Hitomi S, Oishi T, Kondo T, Ebihara T, Funayama Y, et al. Characteristics of bacteremia caused by extended-spectrum beta-lactamase-producing Proteus mirabilis. Journal of Infection and Chemotherapy. 2013; **19**(5):799-805

[21] Li X, Zhao H, Lockatell CV, Drachenberg CB, Johnson DE, Mobley HL. Visualization of Proteus mirabilis within the matrix of urease induced bladder stones during experimental urinary tract infection. Infection and Immunity. 2002; **70**:389-394

[22] Lipsky BA. Urinary tract infections in men. Annals of Internal Medicine. 1989;**110**:138-150

[23] Mbanga J, Masuku S, Luphahla S. Antibiotic resistance patterns and virulence factors of coagulase negative staphylococcus associated with urinary tract infections in Bulawayo Province, Zimbabwe. Journal of Advances in Medicine and Medical Research. 2016; **11**:1-9

[24] McCall J, Hidalgo G, Asadishad B, Tufenkji N. Cranberry impairs selected behaviors essential for virulence in Proteus mirabilis HI4320. Canadian Journal of Microbiology. 2013;**436** (April):430-436

[25] Ofek I, Sharon N, Abraham SN. Bacterial adhesion. Journal of Infection and Chemotherapy. 2011;**715**(11):16-31

[26] Okimoto N, Hayashi T, Ishiga M, Nanba F, Kishimoto M, Yagi S, et al. Clinical features of Proteus mirabilis pneumonia. Journal of Infection and Chemotherapy. 2010;**16**(5):364-366

[27] Olin SJ, Bartges JW. Urinary tract infections treatment/comparative therapeutics. Veterinary Clinics of North America-Small Animal Practice. 2015; **45**(4):721-746

[28] Park S, Kelley KA, Vinogradov E, Solinga R, Weidenmaier C, Misawa Y, et al. Characterization of the structure and biological functions of a capsular polysaccharide produced by *staphylococcus saprophyticus*. Journal of Bacteriology. 2010;**192**(18):4618-4626

[29] Pérez-Lpez FR, Haya J, Chedraui P. Vaccinium macrocarpon: An interesting option for women with recurrent urinary tract infections and other health benefits. The Journal of Obstetrics and Gynaecology Research. 2009;**35**(4):630-639

[30] Probst P. Literature review on the validity of the stepping stones triple P program. Praxis der Kinderpsychologie und Kinderpsychiatrie. 2009;**58**:351-367

[31] Prywer J, Sadowski RR, Torzewska A. Aggregation of struvite, carbonate apatite, and Proteus mirabilis as a key factor of infectious urinary stone formation. Crystal Growth and Design. 2015;**15**(3):1446-1451